ONCC – OCN Exam Practice Questions

Latest 300 Practice Questions with Rationales to easily crack the OCN Exam.

Prof. Rita Carolyn

Dr. Olivia Parks

© 2020-2021

Printed in USA.

Disclaimer

Printed in USA.

Secret of Success – What, Why, How?

What are the Secrets?

- Frequently Asked Questions: Questions are prepared based on the latest curriculum as specified by the ONCC®. The frequently asked questions are given to make you familiarize with the important concepts.
- Sharpen your thinking ability: Our explanation to the practice question will help you to improve your reasoning ability and hence you will be able to answer any type of question with ease.
- Practice, Practice, Practice: More you practice, you get the best out of you. There are 300 practice questions to give you an ample amount of practice.
- No last minute surprise: These practice questions and options are designed in a way that matches the OCN ® Exam so that you don't have a feeling of embarrassment when you take the actual exam.
- More weightage, more exploration: Certain concepts like Symptom Management and Palliative Care, Treatment Modalities are given more weightage in the OCN Exam. Hence we have covered more around these topics which will help you to dive deep in the core concepts and easily pass the exam.

Why this book?

- All the question in this book are prepared and reviewed by Oncology Experts considering the latest curriculum.
- The question and option format exactly matches the actual OCN® Exam conducted by ONCC® so that the test takers will get an idea and experience of attending the exam.
- There are 300 OCN Exam Practice Questions so that you will have an ample amount of practice and gain 100% confidence before

taking the OCN Exam.

- For every question there is an explanation for the correct answer which will make you to understand the concepts clearly, in case if you are not sure of.
- The questions in this book are prepared on the basis of the following curriculum as specified by ONCC®.
  I. Care Continuum - 19%
  II. Oncology Nursing Practice - 17 %
  III. Treatment Modalities - 19%
  IV. Symptom Management and Palliative Care - 23%
  V. Oncologic Emergencies - 12%
  VI. Psychosocial Dimensions of Care - 10%

- More Weightage, More Number of Questions for that concept. The questions are randomly ordered just as in the actual OCN exam to improve thinking ability.

How to pass the exam?

- Try to answer the 300 questions in this book.
- Consider managing time and try to complete 165 questions in Three Hours.
- Correct the questions for which you gave a wrong answer. Understand it from the explanation given in this book.
- Study and explore more on the concepts that you are finding difficult.
- Retake the test until you are familiar with all the 300 questions and getting all the questions right.
- Finally, attend the OCN® Exam with 100% confidence and you will definitely pass the exam.

ALL THE BEST!! YOU WILL SURELY BE AN ONCOLOGY CERTIFIED NURSE !

Table of Contents:

OCN Exam – 300 Practice Questions

OCN Exam – 300 Practice Questions

Question 1: The complications that occur after performing percutaneous lung biopsy is?

a) Pneumonia

b) Pneumothorax

c) Acute or partial collapse of lung or section of lung

d) Building up of fluid between the lung and tissues (Pleural effusion)

Question 2: For managing nausea and vomiting at the end of the life, which of the following complimentary is most likely to be effective?

a) Walking

b) Massage

c) Acupuncture

d) Music therapy

Question 3: The condition that requires treatment by allogeneic stem cell transplant is?

a) Hodgkin Lymphoma

b) Follicular thyroid cancer

c) Chronic Myeloid leukemia

d) Multiple myeloma

Question 4: Advantage of implanted vascular system over a tunneled central vascular system is?

a) Low cost of insertion

b) Reduced risk of infection

c) Short term usage

d) Unlimited ability to access

Question 5: A patient is at the dying stage due to lung cancer. The patient also feels dyspneic. What will the nurse do to make the patient feel less short of breath after finding that his bed is elevated to 45° and also noticed that he is receiving oxygen at 4L / min?

a) The nurse will make the patient lie flat on bed

b) The nurse will turn the airflow of the pedestal fan towards the patient

c) The nurse tries to have a conversation with the patient

d) The nurse informs this to a physician

Question 6: In order to prevent the occurrence of colon cancer, which among the following plays a major role?

a) Daily exercise

b) Diet planning

c) Acetaminophen

d) Vitamins

Question 7: What happens when Mathew gets infused with cryopreserved hematopoietic stem cells?

a) The preservative shall cause a garlic-like taste and odor.

b) This cell infusion happens in a period of 4 days

c) Urine will be pink-tinged at least for a week after infusion

d) IN order to observe the changes, premedication shall not be administered

Question 8: A nurse is working with a patient with terminal illness. Which among the following statement seems to be helpful for her in assisting her patient to reframe hope?

a) "We are always there to help you"

b) "You are still left with more time, don't worry"

c) "Have faith in God, he will save you"

d) "What appears to be more important to you?"

Question 9: A patient continues to work full time even after being fatigue due to radiation therapy. Which will be the most useful suggestion among the following?

a) Start working earlier and complete before the energy levels drop.

b) Keep all the frequently used items under close reach

c) Engage in aerobics workout for 2 hours

d) Involve muscular activity during the worktime

Question 10: At what age prostate specific antigen blood test has to be taken in order to reduce average risk according to American Cancer society Guidelines?

a) 50

b) 20

c) 30

d) 40

Question 11: William is experiencing uncontrolled pain due to bone metastasis. The nurse, the patient and the palliative care are reviewing the plan of care. The above scenario is an example of?

a) Advising

b) Criticize

c) Collaboration

d) Advising

Question 12: Clara returns home to take care of her mother who becomes terminally ill. Her father disagrees with her mother's choice regarding terminal care whereas Clara agrees with her father's choice. They try convincing her mother by applying pressure. This is an example of which theory according to Bowen's Family system?

a) Sentimental

b) Triangular theory

c) Transition

d) Evolution

Question 13: Which of the following below requires immediate assessments?

a) Velcade under the skin

b) Vincristine administered reaches cerebrospinal fluid

c) Asparaginase is given into large muscles

d) Intra peritoneal cisplatin

Question 14: To identify, monitor and improve the effectiveness of oncology nursing care, nurse has collected the data and analyzed it. The above nursing practice exemplifies the?

a) Patient's advocacy standards

b) Collaboration standard

c) Resource utilization standards

d) Collegiality standards

Question 15: Richardson, a 69 year old patient report of sudden increase in temperature of 101°F (38.3°c) and lightheadedness, he received his Chemotherapy a week ago. The nurse identifies that Richard must be dyspneic and diaphoretic. What will be the nurse initial response?

a) Recheck temperature in 2 hours

b) Report to emergency department

c) Call for an ambulance

d) Take paracetamol

Question 16: Persistent fever and chills has been reported by a patient receiving interleukin 2 with neutrophils count of 1500/mm³. What is the representation of these symptoms?

a) Tumor lysis syndrome

b) Septic shock

c) Drug induced reaction

d) Viral infection

Question 17: What will be the choice of treatment for the patient with stage 1 non-small cell lung cancer with impaired pulmonary functions?

a) Removal of lobe of an organ (lobectomy)

b) Removal of Lung (pneumactomy)

c) External beam radiation

d) Platinum based chemotherapy

Question 18: What is the additional role of corticosteroids along with decreasing inflammation?
 a) Reduce anxiety
 b) Improves muscle tone
 c) Stimulate the appetite
 d) Stimulate weight loss

Question 19: Tiara is said to receive her fourth dose of chemotherapy for lung cancer. She experiences nausea suddenly while driving to hospital for her treatment. Which among the following is the type of nausea that Tiara experiences?
 a) Overcoming or Breakthrough
 b) Delayed
 c) Anticipatory
 d) Acute

Question 20: Swelling in the left arm and fingers are reported by patient who underwent mastectomy 3 days ago. While vascular access device is easily flushed, blood return is not obtained. Which case will be suspected among the following?
 a) Thrombosis within the superior Vena Cava
 b) Delayed anaphylactic reaction to paclitaxel
 c) Prolonged dependency of arm positioning
 d) Lymphedema after mastectomy

Question 21: When is adjuvant therapy administered in the case of Breast Cancer?
 a) While locally treating cancer cells with minimal harm to other cells
 b) It doesn't require specific time to be administered and can cure the patient by killing the cancer cells
 c) After the primary therapy in order to increase the chance of disease free survival for a long term.
 d) Before primary therapy, to shrink the tumor that is in operable in its current state

Question 22: Which among the following is said to be the most distressing side effects for the patients undergoing chemotherapy, radiotherapy or biotherapy?

a) Nausea

b) Breathlessness

c) Vomiting

d) Fatigue

Question 23: What type of nausea does the patient receive after 48 hours of chemotherapy?

a) Somatic

b) Delayed

c) Short term

d) Breakthrough

Question 24: Mortality rate can be reduced by using acetyl salicylic acid for which of the following cancer types?

a) Gastrointestinal

b) Malignant neoplasm of testis

c) Cervical

d) Leukemia

Question 25: Which of the following actions characterize the social learning theory?

a) Collaborating to solve problems

b) Trying to goals

c) Trying to imitate other's activity

d) Creating mnemonics

Question 26: The policy and procedure for chemotherapy administration has been reviewed by nurse's manager. In what ways can the ASCO/ ONS Chemotherapy Administration for Safety Standards assist in this process?

a) It provides idea about the professional responsibility of the oncology nurses in chemotherapy administration.

b) It helps in providing description for the oncology nurse jobs

c) The required educational classes for the oncology nurses are being listed

d) The data collection tool regarding the quality improvement are provided

Question 27: What is considered as the most important factor for self-determined closure of life?

a) Honoring wishes of patient regarding end of life care

b) Discharging the patient

c) Stopping the treatment

d) Proceeding with advanced medication

Question 28: Clara has a history of ovarian cancer suddenly reports feeling full after eating small quantity and also experiences an increase in weight. She has noticed an increase of 10 pounds within a week and also states that she is eating less. What will the nurse instruct Clara?

a) Eat small and frequent meals

b) Visit the clinic

c) Report if there is an increase in weight

d) Call when is there is an increase in swelling of ankle.

Question 29: Paclitaxel (PTX), sold under the brand name Taxol among others, is a chemotherapy medication used to treat a number of types of cancer. Harry is administered with the first dose of PTX. He will undergo certain reactions. For which among the following, the nurse should have made the arrangements to treat the Harry?

a) Hypersensitivity reaction

b) Feeling of being in a cold environment with shivering and chills

c) Urinary Retention

d) Vomiting

Question 30: Which among the following clearly denotes the 'purpose of a living will', as taught by the nurse?

a) Appointing surrogate to make medical decisions

b) Making final decision regarding treatment progression

c) Establishment of the patient's desire for care prior to a life threatening illness

d) Acknowledgement of the risk and limiting the recommended therapies

Question 31: Katie with family history of BRCA1 and BRCA2 breast cancer is 20 years old. She enquires about the initiating mammogram. What will the nurse recommend?

a) Having an early mammogram at the age of 35 years

b) Having a breast ultrasound after her first pregnancy

c) Talking with her doctor about advantages and disadvantages of starting the screening earlier.

d) To begin her screening exactly when her family was identified.

Question 32: Mathew complains of itching at the infusion site while administering doxorubicin peripherally. The nurse's initial response to the red streak along with the blood return will be?

a) Continue the drug administration

b) Stop the infusion and flush the line with saline

c) Change the IV site

d) Stop the infusion and instill the antidote

Question 33: In order to reduce anxiety which among the following is suggested?

a) Hyperbaric oxygen therapy

b) Allopathy

c) Meditation

d) Mindfulness-based stress reduction

Question 34: Certain medication can cause increased sedation when administered with opioids. Which of the following medication is the correct option?

a) Narcan

b) Glutocorticoid medication

c) Non steroidal Ibuprofen

d) Chlorpromazine

Question 35: Anticipatory Grief, according to the nurse understanding is?

a) Short term

b) Resolved

c) Unacknowledged

d) Unconscious process

Question 36: Louis receives total body irradiation for hematopoietic stem cell transplant. After one year he reports dullness in vision and ocular sensitivity. What is said to be the cause of above symptoms?

a) Optic neuritis

b) Crossed eye

c) Loss of vision

d) Cataract

Question 37: William has been diagnosed with esophageal cancer. He suddenly reports having difficulty in swallowing and coughing. Which among the following will be considered more by the nurse?
a) Cavity
b) Aspiration
c) Dry mouth
d) Acid reflex

Question 38: Which of the following exemplifies complicated grief as demonstrated by the spouse of the patient who died recently?
a) Seeking out new organization to join
b) Attending the support group for the family of cancer patients
c) Removing all the pictures from the house and refusing to discuss about the descendant
d) Avoiding discussion with hospice service

Question 39: Catherine, suffering from ovarian cancer develops severe nausea ending up vomiting in large volume of fluids. This causes abdominal pain and rigid palpation with diminishing bowel sounds due to little bowel movements. She is not feverish but feels difficulty in breathing. The most preferred diagnosis is:
a) Perforation of gastro intestinal tract
b) Colon Obstruction
c) Small Intestine Obstruction
d) Fecal impactions

Question 40: Michelle is an advanced cancer patient. She is been taken care by her daughter at home. Her daughter states, " No one in my family understand how tiring cooking, cleaning and caring giving can be ". What will be most appropriate solution?
a) Visiting friends
b) Approaching support groups for caregivers
c) Visiting a psychologist
d) Attending motivation camps

Question 41: Which among the following will be the major side effects received by the patient due to the intake of irinotecan?

a) Patchy hair loss

b) Diarrhea

c) Expelling stomach content out of mouth forcefully

d) Constriction of pupil of eye

Question 42: What combines with a mouse to form a cosmetic monoclonal antibody?

a) Pig antibody

b) cow antibody

c) Plant antibody

d) Human antibody

Question 43: Michelle after entering a palliative care underwent a treatment for leukemia that included chemotherapy. The Absolute Neutrophil Count is 526/ mm³, whereas her white blood cells close g is 5300/ mm³. Michelle has higher risk for which among the following options?

a) Fracture

b) Infection

c) Wheezing

d) Hypotension

Question 44: John has been evaluated for chronic leukemia. He has a history for cardiac disease reports of tachycardia and dyspnea. Which of the following blood cell count is most likely to indicate the cause?

a) Absolute neutrophils count - 1700/ mm³

b) White blood cells Count - 2960 mm³

c) Platelet count -1000,000 mm³

d) Level of Hemoglobin - 7.9 g/dl

Question 45: Name the governmental organization which is responsible for the

protection of human subjects and states that when performing studies involving human beings, the researcher must first obtain informed consent, in an easily understandable manner?
a) WHO
b) FDA
c) CDC
d) PAHO

Question 46: Robin was provided with an adequate teaching in chemotherapy and Myelosuppression. He tries to demonstrate with his understanding. Which point is said to initiate his demonstration?
a) Myelosuppression refers to the immune system reaction of the body to a particular medicine.
b) Myelosuppression occurs when there is an elevation in the white blood cell count.
c)Myelosuppression is unintentional before blood transfusion
d) Myelosuppression is a potential side effects to many cancer treatments.

Question 47: A patient is scheduled to receive oxaliplatin. Which of the following denotes that the patient needs additional teaching?
a) Before starting my chemotherapy I'm scheduled to get my first flu shot.
b) I'm going to eat ice chips while receiving chemotherapy in order to avoid mouth sores.
c)I'll call the triage number if I develop fever
d) I have ordered a wig to match my hair color

Question 48: Certain medications tend to interfere with cell membrane bound targets by blocking ligand receptor activation and immune modulation. Which of the following is considered as the interfering medication?
a) Anti-tumor antibiotics
b) Monoclonal antibody
c) Antineoplastic agent
d) Vascular permeability factor

Question 49: The most likely cause of palmar plantar erythrodysesthesia is?

 a) Decreased circulation after infusion

 b) Rupture of capillaries due to pressure and friction

 c) Arranging for an occupational therapy

 d) Over exposure of fast growing skin cells

Question 50: A patient has a visible skin sloughing and tissue breakdown. This is said to occur after Leakage of fluid (Extravasation). Which among the following is appropriate for the above causes?

 a) Application of ice pack

 b) Consultation with plastic surgeon

 c) Administering amoxicillin

 d) Consultation with infectious disease

Question 51:   A patient with lymphoma feels weak while ambulating , dribbling urine and also experience numbness in feet. Which among the following will be the initial suspect by the nurse?

 a) Peripheral neuritis

 b) Endocrine disruptor

 c) Type 1 diabetes

 d) Spinal cord compression

Question 52: The Carcinogenic medication among the following is?

 a) Streptozotocin

 b) Etoposide

 c) Furan

 d) Anthraquinone

Question 53: A patient has been diagnosed with lymphomatous meningitis. Which among the following will be the chemotherapy medication?

a) Vincristine

b) Cytarabine

c) Acyclovir

d) Rifampicin

Question 54: Until which situation should a hospice patient nearing death be offered food and water?

a) As long as the patient wishes to consume food and water.

b) As long as the patient is conscious.

c) Until the patient begins hydration and artificial feeding.

d) Until the patient becomes lethargic.

Question 55: A patient is receiving pain medication throughout the day as the patient was diagnosed with cognitive impairment and metastatic colon cancer. The nurse notes certain actions of patient: This includes short period of hyperventilation, frequent crying, fist clenched and lying rigidly and is increasingly combative. Which among the following matches the nurse suspicion?

a) Increasing mental illness

b) Increasing antibiotics

c) Drowsiness due to pain killers

d) Pain control is not sufficient

Question 56: Among the following, which option can clearly explain the cancer survivorship plan?

a) Outlining about the expected follow up care after the treatment

b) Explaining about the medications

c) Exploring with the hospice care

d) Outlining about the primary therapies received during initial treatments

Question 57: A patient is afebrile with generalized oral erythema, white patches on the palate, xerostomia and lump like sensation while swallowing after one week of chemotherapy. Which among the following can cure the above symptoms?
a) Amoxicillin
b) Pan endoscopy
c) Fluconazole
d) Paracetamol

Question 58: Temozolomide are used for administering certain brain cancer. What will be nurse advice to patient who is about to begin temozolomide medication?
a) Diarrhea is the common side effects
b) Neutropenia occurs after 22 to 28 days of completion
c) Uncommon side effects are nausea and vomiting
d) Weekly monitoring the amount of protein in urine is necessary

Question 59: Harry, with small cell lung cancer has observed the following changes; increase of weight up to 4 pounds, headache and excessive thirst. These are generally the symptoms of?
a) Hemolytic Uremic Syndrome (HUS)
b) Pericardial Tamponade
c) Tumor lysis syndrome
d) SIADH syndrome

Question 60: Proto-oncogenes can be described as?
a) The gene that makes tumor cells back to normal Genes
b) The gene that can provoke abnormal tumor growth
c) A gene that has the ability to become a transformer gene by transforming a normal cell into cancer cell
d) A gene that looks like a normal cell

Question 61: Which of the following cancer type should be screened by 25 year old Michelle with BRCA1 mutation, who also underwent Bilateral Preventative Mastectomies for Breast Cancer?
a) Lymphatic Cancer
b) Brain Cancer
c) Ovarian Cancer
d) Breast Cancer

Question 62: A patient is at her dying stage. Her daughter states that she wishes to do something for her mother's care , but she doesn't know what to do. How can the nurse help the patient's daughter?
a) By showing the daughter about the simple procedures such as mouth care
b) By saying that her presence is enough to make her mother happy
c) By telling her to have a peaceful conversation with her mother
d) By telling her not to disturb her mother

Question 63: Mathew was diagnosed with intractable dyspnea. Even during the end of his life, he didn't find any relief with the traditional intervention. What will be the upcoming step considered by the nurse?
a) Informs the patient about the completion of all the therapies
b) Asks the physician to increase the dosage
c) Calls the anesthetist to increase the dosage of anesthesia
d) Discussing about the Palliative sedation initiated with the team.

Question 64: A patient who has been enrolled in clinical trials has made an informed decision. Which among the following suitably match his informed decision?
a) The physician has explained all these to my family
b) Gained knowledge from cancer blog and came to know about its survival rate
c) Though there is no positive response from family, patient believes the process
d) Physician wouldn't have suggested if it was not suitable.

Question 65: Robert's son insist that he will make all the decision regarding his father's care even though he is alert in making decisions. What will be the appropriate reply of the nurse?

a) To ask his son not to interfere in Robert's decision

b) To arrange a meeting with family members and health care members to discuss patient's wish

c) By allowing his son to make decisions

d) By suggesting motivation groups

Question 66: Which of the following disease can be cured by allogeneic stem cell transplant?

a) Breast Cancer

b) Lymphoma

c) Acute lymphoblastic leukemia

d) Germ cell tumors

Question 67: Which among the following can occur due to the negligence of attending a patient during their end of life?

a) Hopes to recovery

b) Premature death

c) Sense of peace

d) Adequate pain control

Question 68: Robert, a patient with colon cancer underwent a bowel resection with colostomy. He suddenly experiences an abnormal finding on his third postoperative day. Which among the following matches his findings?

a) Moist bright, pink stoma

b) A dull, grey stoma

c) Air in the ostomy appliances

d) Slight stoma bleeding

Question 69: Which of the following medication is given for radiation induced diarrhea?

a) Glutamine

b) Loperamide

c) Erythromycin

d) Cetirizine

Question 70: Cancer patients are generally given opioids to cure severe pains. When a patient suddenly complains about itching (pruritus), what can be done to manage this ?

a) Aspirin

b) Antipyretics

c) Celexa

d) Antihistamines

Question 71: Who is at the greater risk among the following for bone marrow depression after radiation treatment?

a) A 58-year-old patient who is receiving radiation for solitary liver metastasis

b) A 46-year-old patient receiving boost for Lumpectomy site

c) A 25-year-old patient receiving chemotherapy and radiation for Hodgkin lymphoma

d) A 67-year-old patient who is being treated for basal cell carcinoma of face

Question 72: Among the following, which one causes more blisters or is a vesicant?

a) Melphalan

b) Dactinomycin

c) Dalcabazine

d) Topotecan

Question 73: A patient is receiving Fluorouracil and leucovorin for an unresectable T2 N2 M1 adenocarcinoma of the colon. Which among the following is considered as the goal for this treatment?

a) Increase in cellular contact inhibition

b) Promotion of cellular transformation

c) Radio sensitivity promotion

d) Control in cancer growth

Question 74: Which among the following is described as the coping skill that rely on intrapsychic process?
a) Focusses only on problems
b) Focusing on appraisal
c) Focusses on emotion
d) Focusses only on avoidance

Question 75: Michelle, who received cyclophosphamide five years ago for her breast cancer reported about the beginning of bruising and fatigue recently. These symptoms appears to be the suspect for which of the following options?
a) Liver failure
b) Secondary leukemia
c) Cardiomyopathy
d) Leukoencephalopathy

Question 76: In order to screen the malignancy, which among the following tumor marker is used?
a) Prostate-specific antigens
b) CA-125
c) Carcinoembryonic antigen
d) Human chorionic gonadotropin

Question 77: What is the risk factor of development Lymphedema after the surgery for breast cancer?
a) Leukoreduced
b) Low body mass index
c) Axillary node dissection

d) Somatic

Question 78: What type of cancer can be prevented when oral contraceptive pills are consumed for more than 5 years?
a) Endometrial cancer
b) Lung cancer
c) Breast cancer
d) Ovarian cancer

Question 79: The type of cancer that can develop due to excessive use of smokeless tobacco and alcohol is?
a) Lymphatic cancer
b) Lung cancer
c) Gastric cancer
d) Laryngeal cancer

Question 80: When a nurse has the ability to recognize and respect difference in beliefs, values and lifestyle, which among the following will the nurse try to demonstrate?
a) Presentation
b) Non maleficence
c) Protective buffering
d) Cultural competence

Question 81: Before starting the process of chemotherapy, patient has to generally sign a consent form. He has a question regarding the treatment. What will the nurse do now?
a) Ensures of getting the consent form signed and beginning the treatment
b) Begins to administer while explaining the treatment
c) Asks the healthcare general to explain the treatment
d) Addresses patient's concerns before starting the treatment

Question 82: The most effective treatment for the severe pain that is associated with the post herpetic neuropathy is?

a) Dihydromorphinone

b) Extra strength acetaminophen

c) Amitriptyline

d) Propoxyphene

Question 83: The primary source of information by the patient while assessing the level of pain will be?

a) Medication for current pain

b) Self reporting

c) Monitored Vital signs

d) Medical diagnosis

Question 84: Richard has been diagnosed with advanced level of lung cancer. He reports having a rectum disorder, small amount of liquid stools and lower abdominal pain. The nurse will?

a) Withhold all scheduled opioid until bowel function is restored.

b) Provide a non-stimulating laxative

c) Administer oral laxative and probiotic therapy

d) Initiate a bulk forming laxative and force fluids

Question 85: A patient suddenly reports the emergency department of having slurred speech, shuffling gait and Tremors while receiving prochloroperazine. Which of the following causes the above symptoms?

a) Hypocalcemia

b) Heart Attack

c) Extrapyramidal reaction

d) Psychomotor seizure

Question 86: A patient diagnosed with breast cancer was given a dose of IV doxorubicin an anthracycline DNA-binding agent. Soon the patient was observed to be suffering

from symptoms like swelling, redness, itching and vesicles at IV insertion site. The course of action that the nurse should follow after discontinuing the medication is:

a) The nurse should apply some ice and administer dimethyl sulfoxide.

b) The nurse should apply some heat and administer dimethyl sulfoxide.

c) The nurse should apply some ice and administer dexrazoxane.

d) The nurse should apply some heat and administer dexrazoxane.

Question 87: After a loop electrosurgical excision procedures, what information will the nurse provide to the patient?

a) To avoid inserting anything into the vagina for 4 weeks

b) To expect extreme fatigue for several months

c) To Sit upright most of the time

d) To begin an exercise program to reduce weight gain

Question 88: In order to decrease the sleep disturbances, which of the following can be suggested?

a) Setting a comfortable bedroom temperature

b) Watching movies prior to bedtime.

c) Requesting the healthcare provider to stop treatment

d) Stretching in bed and doing moderate exercise

Question 89: What is the most common cause of lung cancer?

a) Exposure to direct or secondary tobacco smoke.

b) Genetic mutation.

c) Exposure to ultraviolet rays from the sun.

d) Exposure to chemical waste.

Question 90: Who has a higher risk of skin breakdown?

a) A patient with hyperpigmentation

b) A patient with decreased sensory perception

c) A patient with decreased serum albumin level

d) Higher mobilized patient

Question 91: Which among the following is said to be the suitable integrative modality for the patient who has pain with a platelet count of 12000/mm³?
a) Chemotherapy
b) Massage
c) Reiki therapy
d) Acupuncture

Question 92: What is best approach while helping a dying patient in completing a life review?
a) By asking question without any hesitation in order to acquire more knowledge
b) By asking regular question
c) By having a comfortable conversation with the patient
d) By making a formal conversation with the family members

Question 93: Breast cancer survivor suddenly weeps to a nurse saying that she didn't expect that lymphedema would happen to her. How will the nurse react the patient?
a) By allowing the patient to express her feelings
b) By assuring the quick recovery of lymphedema
c) By teaching the prevention methods of lymphedema recurrence
d) By taking a recent history to identify the occurrence of lymphedema

Question 94: Which of the following principles does advanced directives are based upon?
a) Kindness
b) Autonomy
c) Justice
d) Truthfulness

Question 95: A patient with glioblastomas has been receiving radiation therapy. Which among the following would be the statement mentioned by the patient after understanding the teachings?

a) ' I shall avoid hair wash '

b) ' I can now stop taking steroids '

c)' I might experience permanent hair loss '

d) ' I shouldn't worry having a head ache. '

Question 96: **Which among the following statement correctly explains about the use of spouse as a translator for non-English speaking patient?**

a) Translation by spouse can generally increase the patient's confidence level

b) Translation by the patients spouse is not recommended

c) Translation is allowed only when the spouse clear a qualification test

d) Translation is allowed only when the professional is not available

Question 97: **What will be the first step in oncology clinical setting using evidence based practices?**

a) Assess the patient need to define the problem

b) Using a medical model to explain the problems

c) Adding all the changes in care to experience the outcome

d) Before literature research, define the patient's outcome.

Question 98: **Which of the following is the primary measure to prevent cancer?**

a) Guaiac fecal occult blood test

b) Usage of sunscreen

c) Systemic estrogens therapy

d) Self-examination of testicle

Question 99: **The following are the symptoms of a patient suffering from stage IV Lung Cancer; Difficulty in differentiating between anginal pain (progressive dyspnea), facial swelling; swelling of neck, arms,hands and thorax due to the fluid from the tissue; Distended jugular,temporal and arm veins; disturbance in vision; headache and disorientation (altered mental status). The diagnosis for the above symptoms are:**

a) Superior Vena Cava Syndrome (SVCS)

b) Lung embolism

c) Compression of Spinal Cord

d) Syndrome for Inappropriate secretion of Anti-Diuretic Hormone(SIADH)

Question 100: For muscle invasive bladder cancer which among the following is said to be the primary goal?
a) Preventing the development to brain
b) Preparing the body for chemotherapy
c) Reducing the surgery time
d) Preserving the bladder function

Question 101: Which of the following conditions are included in Myeloablation for transplanting stem cell?
a) Growth analysis
b) Nutritional analysis
c) High dose chemotherapy
d) Retrograde surgical intervention

Question 102: Cherry is a survivor of Malignant Melanoma. She has completed her treatment one year ago, but still complains about tiredness. Which among the following stimulants does the nurse foretell?
a) Lorazepam
b) Darbepoetin Alfa
c) Pegfilgrastim
d) Methylphenidate

Question 103: What has to be done when Robin reports of yellow, crusted papules and itching of shoulder after a targeted therapy?
a) Dilute hot bath water with half strength Dakin's solution
b) Apply lotion with Dimethicone
c) Using a moisturizer containing retinoid twice a day
d) Apply aloe Vera on the affected region

Question 104: Jonas, 62 years old patient with CD33 positive acute myeloid leukemia has a left ejection fraction of 40% during first relapse. What is the treatment suggested for Jonas?

a) All trans retinoic acids

b) Gemtuzumab ozogamicin

c) Cytosine arbinoside

d) Intravenous drug Rituximab

Question 105: In what ways does the cancer cell differ from the ordinary cells?

a) Cancer cells divide only when the older cells are destroyed

b) Cancer cells migrate to the neighboring locations and tissues

c) Ordinary cells generally reside in new areas

d) Ordinary cells doesn't allow contact with the other cells

Question 106: Robert, a 19 year old patient diagnosed with testicular cancer fears about his potency to conceive children as he will be receiving cisplatin and pelvic radiation. What will be suggested for Robert by the nurse?

a) Cryopreservation after completion of cisplatin treatment

b) Preserving the sperm before initiating the treatment

c) Sexual counseling throughout the treatment

d) After the completion of the treatment, sildenafil is given to patient before engaging into sexual activity.

Question 107: NIOSH approved respirator should be worn for which of the following activity?

a) Penetrating an intravenous bag

b) While handling bodily fluids

c) Cleaning hazardous drug spill

d) While Administering an IV chemotherapeutic agent

Question 108: What will be the common adverse effect of a patient diagnosed with prostate cancer when treated with diethylstilbestrol?

a) Pneumonia

b) Gynecomastia

c) Arthritis

d) Bowel obstruction

Question 109: A patient who is at the dying state experiences delirium. Medication that can manage this symptom will be?

a) Cetirizine

b) Haloperidol

c) Aprepitant

d) Paracetamol

Question 110: William suddenly got provoked with a doubt while Docetaxel was infused. He asked the nurse why dexamethasone is prescribed. The nurse responds by saying that it prevents ?

a) Fatigue

b) Sudden uncontrolled electric disturbances

c) Fluid retention

d) Anorexia nervosa

Question 111: What is the major benefit of survivorship care plan?

a) It allows the patient to make discussion with their oncologist after the completion of treatment.

b) It will be easier to monitor patient regarding side effects

c) It allows the patient to have medication during chemotherapy

d) It provides a clear idea about the care and surveillance after treatment

Question 112: A patient with cancer experiences an erectile dysfunction. Which type of intervention is more likely to assist the patient?

a) Psychotherapy

b) Kegel exercise

c) Herbal dietary fibers

d) Oral phosphodiesterase type 5 inhibitors

Question 113: How can the points be focused on the adults who have low literacy rate, during the cancer education programs?

a) Explaining the process with cartoon type illustration.

b) By providing information in the form of quiz

c) Explaining with medical term for better understanding

d) Repeating the same message in different form.

Question 114: William experiences extensive metastasis. He says, " I don't want any treatment. Anyways I'm going to die let me spend my time with my family". What will be the intervention of the nurse?

a) " You will definitely feel better tomorrow"

b) " Would you like to discuss about the hospice service?"

c)" Completing your treatment is more important"

d) " Did you discuss this with your support group?'

Question 115: Which of the following should the patient follow while receiving intraperitoneal cisplatin?

a) Nothing has to be taken orally for 12 hours prior to treatment

b) Changing the position frequently while receiving medication

c) Medication has to be received under fluoroscopy

d) Medication has to be cold

Question 116: What is the common side effect of palanosetron?

a) Hiccups

b) Itchiness

c) Constipation

d) Disturbance in mental ability

Question 117: Which among the following is the symptom exhibited by the newly diagnosed acute myeloid leukemia?

a) Palpitation

b) Headache

c) Petechiae

d) Pruritus

Question 118: William is taking opioids for pain management. He reported of increased constipation and has started bowel retaining. What is said to be the best time to assist him to sit on a toilet or commode to initiate bowel evacuation?

a) Exactly before going to sleep

b) Early in the morning

c) About half an hour after meal

d) Whenever the patient urges to defecate

Question 119: Michele is using fentanyl patches to control her pain caused due to ovarian cancer. She reports the nurse regarding the following symptoms; Difficulty in urinating and able to pass only small amount of urine. Bladder is not distended and has bilateral pain in the flank areas. Recent blood test reports shows slight hyperkalemia and is afebrile. These symptoms are due to?

a) Infection in bladder

b) Cervical cancer

c) Obstruction in upper urinary tract

d) Side effects caused by the intake of opioids

Question 120: What will be the primary nursing intervention of the patient who develops grade 3 peripheral neuropathy?

a) Monitor serum electrolytes

b) Obtain an order for corticosteroids

c) To teach about safe home environment

d) Recommend for increased narcotic analgesia

Question 121: In order to determine acute changes in nutritional status and also to monitor the dietary status of patient with cachexia, test are generally taken. Which of the following is most commonly monitored?
a) Transferrin
b) Albumin and Globulin
c) Prealbumin
d) Albumin

Question 122: A patient with prostate cancer experiences metastasis. Which among the following is said to metastasize frequently?
a) Brain
b) Liver
c) Bone
d) Lung

Question 123: A Fluorouracil based chemotherapy combination has been administered to Ron, who has been employed as a landscaper. Which among the following symptom is most likely to occur?
a) Pulmonary toxicity
b) Gouty arthritis
c)Accumulation of fluid in lower limbs
d) Photosensitivity

Question 124: A gay man is at the dying stage because of leukemia. He asked the hospice not to allow his parents to meet him in his room as his parents didn't accept his lifestyle or his partner. What will be best action done by the nurse?
a) The nurse can ask his parents to leave a message as they are not allowed to meet him
b) The nurse can request the patient to meet his parents
c) The nurse informs his parents about his unwillingness to meet them
d) The nurse can talk with the hospice

Question 125: Rosie, a 60-year-old obese diabetic patient is experiencing bleeding due to post menopause. Which of the following type of cancer is likely to occur in Rosie?

a) Fallopian tube

b) Cervical

c) Ovary

d) Endometrial

Question 126: Restlessness, insomnia, diarrhea, heart palpitations, and irritability are the reactions expressed by newly diagnosed cancer patient. Patient also gets nervous and worried and asks for some medication for nerves. What will be the best response from the nurse?

a) Instructs the patient to ask for a sedative from the physician.

b) Informs the patient about the initiation of treatment

c) Ask the patient to explain his feelings further

d) Assure that the reason is due to cancer diagnosis

Question 127: Robin experiences persistent depressive disorder (dysthymic behavior) for several weeks. What should the nurse assess initially?

a) Depression

b) Bowel Habits

c) Recurrence of disease

d) Cognitive learning

Question 128: Mild ascites along with increase in weight and early satiety were the complaints reported by the recently diagnosed lung cancer patient. There is a possibility of developing malignant ascites. Which among the following improves the risk?

a) Renal disease

b) Diabetes

c) Pulmonary Disease

d) Diverticulitis

Question 129: What will be the initiation taken by the nurse when a patient complains about urticaria and pruritus while getting paclitaxel infused?

a) Administering diphenhydramine

b) Obtaining vital signs and monitor patients

c) Applying ice packs to the affected region.

d) The infusion of the medication has to be stopped

Question 130: The patient has sudden dyspnea, wheezing, hypotension, throat and face swelling during the administration of chemotherapeutic agent intravenously. What will be the initial action of the nurse?

a) To stop administering oxygen

b) To decrease antihistamine

c) To discontinue the administering of chemotherapeutic agent

d) To increase administering epinephrine

Question 131: Certain population is at the risk for the under treatment of pain during their end of the life. Which among the following correctly matches?

a) Younger adults

b) Elderly people

c) Diabetic patient

d) Men

Question 132: Which of the following is considered as a modal quality of cancer treatment regarding surgery?

a) It causes less toxicity when used along with chemotherapy

b) It is considered as the only treatment that the patient requires

c) It is used as a palliative measure to relieve symptoms

d) It aims to remove only a portion of tumor

Question 133: The cells from which oligodendroglia tumors originate maintains the function of ?

a) Synovial fluid

b) Pericardial fluid

c) Myelin sheath

d) Cell body

Question 134: A patient refuses to take opioids stating that even pain is a part of life. What will be the nurse response to this statement?

a) Exploring the meaning of pain with the patient

b) Schedule a visit with CanSurmount volunteer

c) Requesting an evaluation from the pain service

d) Referring pain to chaplain

Question 135: Richard is learning about patient controlled analgesia (PCA) pump from his nurse. Even though his nurse taught him the process at least for 3 times, he kept asking the same doubts repeatedly. The nurse also provides Richard with a pamphlet but he doesn't look at it at all. He says that he can't understand anything by looking at the pamphlet and doesn't know what to do next. What will be the next step taken by the nurse?

a) By allowing the patient to practice with the kit

b) By asking another nurse to teach him

c) By suggesting other alternative methods

d) By starting her teaching after some rest time

Question 136: A patient has developed a wheel and pain at peripheral IV site during infusion of Doxorubicin. Which among the following is said to be an appropriate intervention?

a) Heat application

b) Administering mesnex

c) Applying hydrocortisone

d) Administering dexrazoxane

Question 137: Charles has been diagnosed with invasive ductal adenocarcinoma of pancreas. Upon diagnosis, the disease most likely:

a) Metastatic to Cartilage

b) Remains without spreading to other body parts

c) Demonstrates the spread to liver

d) Displays the widespread fat globules

Question 138: Which among the following reference will assist the nurse in determining the characteristics and safe handling precautions of medicine about which the nurse is concerned as being hazardous?

a) The Joint Commission Hospital Patient Safety Goals

b) NIOSH List of Antineoplastic and Other Hazardous Drug in Healthcare Setting

c) National Comprehensive Cancer Network Clinical Practice Guidelines in Oncology

d) The Joint Commission Hospital Patient Safety Goals

Question 139: For which of the practice standard of oncology nursing society should the nurse demonstrate behavioral consent for taking oncology certified nurse examination?

a) Ethical behavior

b) The extent to which the healthcare services are provided to the individual

c) Performance review

d) Professional performance

Question 140: While treating with interleukin-2, which among the following is said to respond?

a) Advanced testicular cancer

b) Metastatic melanoma

c) Accumulation of abnormal B lymphocyte

d) Urothelial carcinoma

Question 141: Which among the following is considered as the most important criteria for selecting the patient to participate in the phase 2 clinical trial?

a) The patient must have physiological diseases

b) The patient must have an adequate performance status

c) The patient should not be exposed to any chemotherapy treatment before.

d) The patient exhausted all approved treatments

Question 142: William requires chronic platelet transfusions may develop antibodies and require further products to be:

a) Low body mass index

b) Reduced volume

c) Delayed

d) Leukoreduced

Question 143: Unilateral orchiectomy was scheduled for William who has testicular cancer. He enquires the nurse about his reproduction activities. What will be the response of nurse to William?

a) 50% reduction in fertility

b) Azoospermia

c) No change in fertility

d) Oligospermia

Question 144: William, a patient with prostate cancer administers oxycodone orally for the relief from pain every 4 hours. A Nurse, while paying a home visit finds that there has been no bowel movement with constant and dull back pain for the past 3 days. These symptoms are likely to indicate?

a) Adverse effect of oxycodone

b) Excess abdominal fluid (Ascites)

c) Hypocalcemia

d) Impending spinal cord compression

Question 145: Adjunct treatment option for neuropathy has been suggested by the thalidomide receiving patient. The suggestion given by the nurse based on the current evidence would be ?

a) Glutathione

b) Anticonvulsant medication Lamotrigine

c) Fish oil

d) Acupuncture

Question 146: What type of chemotherapy induced nausea does the patient experience after four days of chemotherapy?

a) Acute

b) Prolonged

c) Delayed

d) Refractory

Question 147: Weight loss, abdominal pain and diarrhea are some of the symptoms reported by Harry who is 70 years old. He also reported that these symptoms often interrupts his sleep. Harry's brother was recently diagnosed for prostate cancer. What will the nurse suspect?

a) Spastic colon

b) Klinefelter syndrome

c) Carcinoid syndrome

d) Neurofibromatosis

Question 148: After two weeks of chemotherapy, a patient reports bleeding gums and increased bruises even though the patient has normal platelet count. What is appropriate intervention to be done by the nurse?

a) Review the patient's medical report

b) Suggest the patient to have iron rich food

c) Reassure the patient that this symptoms will reduce after few days

d) Review the patient's history for prior treatment with ionizing radiation

Question 149: Paresthesia and dysesthesia (abnormal sensation) to hands, feet and mouth are caused by which of the following medication?

a) Ifex

b) Busulfan

c) Ifosfamide

d) Oxaliplatin

Question 150: Michelle, a patient has a negative result for BRCA mutation but her sister Rosie has a positive result. What kind of emotion does Michelle exhibit when she says with tears," I was always the troublesome kid"?

a) Survivor Guilt

b) Siblings rivalry

c) Transmitter guilt

d) Reactive Depression

Question 151: Radiation therapy is given to the patient with a tumor on the floor of the mouth. What advice is given to the patient?

a) Avoid using topical anesthetic

b) Avoid consuming alcohol

c) Avoid using less spices

d) Consume only less fluid everyday

Question 152: The nurse observes a raised pearly lesions on the patient's upper chest after completing the physical examination. Which among the following shows the above symptom?

a) Carcinoid syndrome

b) Pneumonitis

c) A basal cell carcinoma

d) Lung cancer

Question 153: Charles, a 21 year old cancer patient suddenly withdrew from college due to cancer resurrection. His family informs the nurse about his mood swings and refusal to meet his friends. What will be strategy achieved by the nurse initially?

a) Re enrolling in college courses

b) Clinical trial participation

c) Recognizing self-destructive behavior

d) Maintaining open communication

Question 154: Which among the following should the nurse focus while considering rehabilitation principle in a cancer patient?

a) Encouraging more rest periods

b) Focusing more on disabilities

c) Develop group goals

d) Emphasize capabilities

Question 155: Mathew, a 78 year old patient has been diagnosed with prostate cancer and cardiovascular disease. He has been administered with naproxen twice a day along with a daily dose of acetylsalicylic acid. What will be the instruction given to the patient?

a) Consulting the physician regarding the addition of cytoprotectants

b) About the increase in swelling during evening times

c) Consumption of medicine only in the empty stomach

d) To consume every medicine with proper time interval

Question 156: What is the most effective team size while developing multidisciplinary team?

a) 12- 16 members

b) 1- 5 members

c) 12- 15members

d) 11- 20 members

Question 157: Persistent nausea, muscle cramps, weakness, and paresthesia of the fingers two days after receiving the first cycle of chemotherapy are the symptoms reported by the patient with Lymphatic cancer or lymphoma. Which among the following is experienced by the patient?

a) Tumor lysis syndrome

b) Syndrome of anti-diuretic secretion hormone

c) Hypercalcemia

d) Disseminated intra vascular coagulation/ consumptive coagulopathy

Question 158: Before initiating the opioid therapy for Pain control, what order does the nurse anticipate initially?

a) Treating occasional constipation

b) Stimulant laxative

c) Suppositories

d) Bulk laxative (Metamucil)

Question 159: According to the Buddhist tradition, they believe that a deceased person's body should not be disturbed for at least four hours. The most likely reason behind this might be:

a) The person might have been diagnosed with an infectious disease and they might need some time to dispose the body properly.

b) They believe that a soul needs some time to leave off the body and be at peace.

c) The patient's family might need some time to cope-up with the patient's loss.

d) The patient's family may need some time to do the final rituals of the patient for his well-being in the afterlife.

Question 160: Among the following, which phase requires data monitoring committee

for clinical trials?

a) 5

b) 3

c) 2

d) 1

Question 161: Mark who has colon mesothelioma has been scheduled for chemotherapy which is to be administered in the peritoneal space. Which is the type of device through which Mark attends his chemotherapy?

a) Intraventricular catheter reservoir (Ommaya reservoir)

b) Large diameter silicon port implantation

c) Insertion of central catheter peripherally

d) Arterial Catheter

Question 162: The ethnic group that has high risk for developing cancer in Male is?

a) Pacific islanders

b) Asian Americans

c) African Americans

d) White Americans

Question 163: List the two types of cancer for which hormone therapy is effective?

a) Liver and lymphoma

b) Breast and prostate

c) Leukemia and breast

d) Liver and prostate

Question 164: Among the following which is considered as the risk factor for the treatment related to pneumonitis?

a) Usage of steroids continuously

b) Lowering the concentration of oxygen therapy

c) For age less than 60 years

d) Mantle field radiation

Question 165: Why are certain tumor cells described as undifferentiated cells?
a) Because they grow at a faster rate
b) Because they resemble normal cells
c) Because they don't grow
d) Because they remain in same position

Question 166: What will be the response of the nurse when enquired about the risk of Lymphedema after undergoing breast conservation surgery with sentinel lymph node biopsy procedure and radiation?
a) If Lymphedema guidelines are followed then there will be no occurrence
b) If there is no development in the first year, then there is no development in the progressive years.
c) Although the risk is low precaution has to be taken
d) There is no occurrence of Lymphedema after sentinel lymph node procedure

Question 167: A patient named Bill Bezos has been experiencing delirium. He is also suffering from marked confusions and hallucinations. Bill believes that the nurse is her daughter and he asks her if everyone at home is alright. The most appropriate reply for the nurse would be?
a) " I am your nurse Mary Lisa".
b) " Please stop dreaming bill".
c) "Yes, everyone is fine back home".
d) "I am not your child'.

Question 168: How will the nurse react when the patient says, " I wanted God to help me to cure cancer but I'm worried that he let me get cancer as I was so angry on him?"
a) The nurse offers contact of a social worker to counsel patient
b) The nurse explains that the religion is not a part of the nursing expertise therefore gives the contact of patient's clergy person.
c) The nurse explores patient's feeling of anger and abandonment
d) The nurse offers sleeping pill for the patient so that the patient can rest enough to

overcome such thoughts.

Question 169: Michelle, a patient with breast cancer asks the nurse during counselling, "How long should I wait for my pregnancy after chemotherapy?". The nurse replies by saying,
a) You should wait at least one year
b) No delay is necessary
c) Infertility is said to be the permanent side effect of the therapy
d) Pregnancy will increase the chances of recurrence

Question 170: Harry has been diagnosed with stage IV lung cancer and brain metastasis. He has been receiving whole brain radiation therapy. Which of the following is considered as the intent of the treatment?
a) Palliative
b) Prevention of disease (prophylactic)
c) Curative
d) Boosting immune response (adjuvant)

Question 171: Among the following condition of the cancer patient, who is most likely to experience sexual dysfunction?
a) A patient and partner who schedule time for their sexual activity.
b) A patient who has a history of marital discord
c) A female patient with hypertension
d) A young and newly married patient

Question 172: Janet is newly diagnosed with cancer so she has quit her job and other social activity. What will be the nurse's response to Janet?
a) By asking about the activity she enjoyed the most before starting treatment
b) By asking her to focus on her cancer
c) By encouraging her that she will be able to join after treatment
d) By saying that her friends would be proud of Janet being a brave overcoming cancer

Question 173: Doxorubicin is given to patient through peripheral IV catheter. The patient reports burning at the site without any swelling. What will be the initial action of the nurse?

a) Administration is continued while observing the site

b) Patient's arm reposition

c) Stop the administration of the drug

d) 10 ml of 0.9% of normal saline is flushed

Question 174: The actions that require the input source from every individual of the multidisciplinary team is?

a) Improving pain medications

b) Skin care routines

c) Development of care plan

d) Medications for healthy appetite

Question 175: What action will the nurse take if the family members of the dying patient disagree on placing the feeding tube?

a) Encourages the family to go through similar cases

b) Explains that only the management can make decisions

c) Meets the family to discuss the goals of care

d) Communicates with the social workers to begin the process

Question 176: The role of proto oncogene is to ?

a) Causes programmed cell death

b) Promote cell division

c) Stimulate angiogenesis

d) Promote cell division

Question 177: Spouse of the patient has been receiving benefits through the Hospice Medicare Benefits. Which of the following is expressed after proper understanding of the teaching?

a) " The coverage of curative chemotherapy will continue for several months"

b) " This benefit can only control the patient's pain"

c)" I will call my hospice provider before taking my spouse to the emergency department"

d) " Curative chemotherapy treatment coverage shall continue for several months"

Question 178: The state of having lost their significant person is generally termed as?

a) Guilt

b) Happiness

c) Grief

d) Bereavement

Question 179: Robert is allowed to participate in phase 2 clinical trial though he doesn't know to speak English. The patient's grandson wishes to translate to receive informed consent. Which of the following will be the most appropriate option?

a) Having an interpreter to translate with grandson present

b) Allowing grandson to act as an interpreter

c) Language barrier shall disallow patient's participation.

d) Having an interpreter to translate without grandson.

Question 180: Continuous Quality Improvement, or CQI, is a management philosophy that organizations use to reduce waste, increase efficiency, and increase internal (meaning, employees) and external (meaning, customer) satisfaction. Which among the following is the core concept of CQI?

a) Problems relate to processes and variations in process lead to variations in results

b) Systemic process improvement to be successful

c) Institute organizational transparency

d) Change emanates from the top

Question 181: What will the next step of the nurse after administering long acting morphine tablet instead of long acting oxycodone?

a) Call the risk management department to guide the documentation

b) Monitoring the patient for next 8 hours continuously

c) Stopping the further medication of patient

d) Notify the patient and the physician of error

Question 182: Shortness of breath, fatigue and swelling are reported by the patient who has been scheduled for chemotherapy. Physical assessment reveals neck vein distention, edema of the hands, tachycardia, and cyanosis. What will be instructed by the nurse to the patient before calling a physician?

a) Lie flat and prepares the patient for thoracotomy
b) Sit up and anticipates an order for a chest-x-ray
c) Lie flat and prepares the patient for echocardiogram
d) Sit up and begins chemotherapy infusion

Question 183: Marcus with recurrent cancer is deteriorating due to his old age. His children are not sure of his wishes. Discussion with family and friends helps?

a) To focus on family desire for the patient
b) To find the available and appropriate option
c) To divide the property of the patient equally
d) To agree with the hospital ethics teams

Question 184: 5 mg of immediate release oxycodone is released 5 to 6 times daily when Mr.Smith receives 10mg of Sustained release Oxycodone for every 12 hours. Which of the following order has to be requested for the best adjustment in pain medication regimens?

a) 10 mg of sustained-release oxycodone every 8 hours
b) 30 mg of immediate-release oxycodone every 6 hours
c) 30 mg of sustained-release oxycodone every 12 hours
d) 10 mg of immediate-release oxycodone every 12 hours

Question 185: Thrombocytopenia is referred as the decrease in the number of circulating platelets below 100, 000/mm^3.What has to be taught to the patient to avoid the risk due to thrombocytopenia?

a) Walking barefoot
b) Having a haircut

c) Using soft bristled toothbrush

d) High fiber food consumption

Question 186: **Ronnie Reacts by displaying maladaptive response for the diagnosis of cancer. This indicates that Ronnie is?**

a) Fighting the treatment for his children

b) Lowering his concentration on treatment

c) Feeling abandoned by God

d) Focusing to live in the present moment

Question 187: **A Lymphedema patient was reported using reflexology for the affected arm who was seen in the outpatient clinic. What will the nurse enquire?**

a) Recommending to use compression sleeve

b) Can u provide me with more information on this technique?

c) Lymphedema will subside over time

d) This method has a promising cure in clinical trials

Question 188: **The recently developed teaching booklet about immunotherapy was evaluated. It indicates that there is no increase in the group of patient's understanding about immunotherapy in the booklet. Which among the following has been considered as prominent principle?**

a) Verbal teaching increases the learning efficiency

b) Teaching is more effective when it responds to the need identified by the patient

c) The effectiveness of the learning is determined by the teaching methodology

d) Guideline for evaluation is provided depending on teacher's expectation

Question 189: **Rihanna has been diagnosed with breast cancer. She has been receiving radiation therapy. She reports to her nurse over her decreased libidos. What will be the appropriate nursing interventions?**

a) Recommend look good feel better programs

b) Gives instructions about the vaginal dilators

c) Explores patient's feeling regarding sexular activity

d) Reassures the patient that it will return

Question 190: A patient who is nearing death , was noticed with an audible gurgling during breathing by a nurse. How can the nurse explain the sound to the patient's family members visiting the patient?

a) " This sound is normal for any patient at this stage"

b) " Due to fluid accumulation, congestion in throat and lungs occur"

c)" He is at his end stage"

d) " These are the side effects of his medications"

Question 191: Which of the following should be worn by the nurse as a protective equipment while injecting intravesical mitomycin?

a) One pair of powdered nitrile glove

b) A Plastic face shield

c) A laboratory gown

d) Shoe covers

Question 192: While discussing the ethical principles regarding the side effects of chemotherapy to a staff, the nurse tries to put forth her point saying that positive effects should bring more good effects than the negative effects bringing bad. Which of the following ethical principle is this related?

a) Justice

b) Non harming or inflicting least harm.

c) Beneficence

d) Autonomy

Question 193: Which among the following is developed as secondary malignancy in patients who have Hodgkin lymphoma?

a) Ovarian cancer

b) Skin cancer

c) Colorectal cancer

d) Leukemia

Question 194: Among the following option, which is the best mediation to increase the patient's adherence for taking oral chemotherapy at home?

a) In order make the patient take over the counter medicine for nausea

b) It will be easier for the patient to take up the refill when the supply runs out during the next appointment

c) It will be easier to monitor the patient regarding the side effects

d) In order to make the patient feel convenient about taking a double dose in case if the patient missed the medication

Question 195: Oral mucositis is caused by?

a) Fluorouracil

b) Interleukin 2

c) Paracetamol

d) Amoxicillin

Question 196: Which of the following is most likely to treat opioid related constipation?

a) Mineral oil

b) Bowel stimulants

c) Laxative

d) Tea tree oil

Question 197: When the adult children of the patient who passed away approaches the nurse expressing the feelings, then the nurse can provide support to the family by?

a) Validating these as normal feelings of grief

b) Encouraging a family conference

c) Validating the necessity of counseling for these feelings

d) Encouraging discussion with Physician

Question 198: What will be the duration of nadir to occur, after completing the chemotherapy treatment cycle?

a) 1- 3 weeks

b) 2- 5 weeks

c) 3 weeks

d) 7- 10 days

Question 199: Darbepoetin Alfa has been administered for the patient with advanced stage of breast cancer. Which among the following are the risk associated according to patient's understanding?

a) Improvement in anemia and the disease may progress

b) Improvement of anemia causing less risk

c) Risk are only for those who have large tumors

d) With each injection the risk of bleeding and infections get doubled.

Question 200: A newly diagnosed patient enquires the nurse about all the tests for clinical staging as suggested by doctor. Which among the following will be the answer given by nurse according to her knowledge regarding staging?

a) Compares the result across population

b) Assess usual spreading pattern of cancer

c) Evaluates the extend of local and potential metastatic disease

d) Predicts response to treatment

Question 201: Harry, Colon cancer survivor wishes to change his job. But he fears that he won't be able to receive his insurance due to his cancer history. What will the nurse advice?

a) Refer him to a support group

b) Encourages him to speak with a lawyer

c) Inform him about the Americans with Disabilities Act of 1990

d) Provides contact of National Coalition of cancer survivorship.

Question 202: A patient reports of difficulty in doing the regular chores due to dyspnea after completing chemotherapy and radiation therapy for mediastinum. Which of the following is the result of the above symptoms?

a) Lung Cancer

b) Brain cancer

c) Deconditioning

d) Pneumonitis

Question 203: Robert has reported the following symptoms; a temperature of 102°F (38.7°C), cough, neutrophils count of 200/ mm³ and tenderness around the central venous catheter. What will be the step taken by the nurse?

a) Obtain chest X-ray

b) Initiate colloidal intravenous fluids

c) Obtain blood cultures from 2 sites

d) Administer acetaminophen 500mg.

Question 204: The need for descending colostomy has been discussed with John who has Colorectal cancer. What will be the position of stoma?

a) Left lower quadrant

b) Just below the waistline

c) Left upper quadrant

d) Right lower quadrant

Question 205: For which of the following diagnosis, Asparaginase has been demonstrated as a clinical response?

a) Hairy-cell leukemia

b) Acute lymphocytic leukemia

c)Brain cancer

d) Non-small cell cancer

Question 206: Among the following statements made by the patient which of the following options correctly indicate the need of education for prevention of infection?

a) I won't allow meeting my grandchildren when they are sick.

b) I do not want to get an influenza shot until all my chemotherapy is finished

c) I'll be more careful while washing hands after gardening.

d) I'll keep my wound dressing supplies in a closed container

Question 207: Rochelle, a 34 year old patient has been diagnosed with breast cancer. Counseling has been given to Rochelle and her partner William regarding contraception before chemotherapy. Which of the following statement ensures adequate understanding by the couple?

a) "Hormone pills are the easiest and the safest method of birth control."
b) " I don't have to worry about birth control before receiving chemotherapy"
c)"I will call my gynecologist to discuss about having my tubes tied."
d) "I will agree to use birth control pills or a reliable barrier method as recommended by my physician."

Question 208: While providing assistance in resolving patient's spiritual pain during end stage, what will be the prior intervention made by the nurse?

a) Mobilizing patient's support system
b) Acknowledge the legitimacy of the patient's pain
c) Encouraging patient to reduce focus on the issues
d) Encouraging reflection of random life events

Question 209: The treatment plan is outlined during initial evaluation and this includes amputation of leg. Suddenly the patients begins to scream and cry saying that he need to walk, play and run with his little children. The response of the nurse will be?

a) The chance of dying is higher if we don't receive amputation.
b) It sounds like you fear your treatment plan, tell me what you know about it
c) The psychiatric nurse will help you cope with the amputation.
d) After fitting with prosthesis, many patients feel better.

Question 210: A patient receiving a high dosage of methotrexate is administered with intravenous fluid containing sodium bicarbonate. This is done to:

a) Protect against Vomiting
b) Eliminate the leucovorin rescue needs
c)Maintain alkaline urine

d) Reduce sensitivity to reaction

Question 211: William, while recieving chemotherapy has developed tissue swelling in the mouth which increases his mouth pain while brushing with toothpaste. What can be suggested as the alternative brushing method in order to avoid pain?
a) Standard mouthwash
b) Salt water
c) Lidocaine based mouth wash
d) Only water

Question 212: Which antiemetic causes potential side effects such as headache and constipation?
a) Zofran (odansetron)
b) Phenothiazine
c) Aprepitant
d) Amoxicillin

Question 213: Anti Nausea medications are generally administered to the patients to prevent anticipatory nausea due to chemotherapy. Which of the following is said to be the right time to medicate the patient ?
a) Daily during chemotherapy
b) Before Chemotherapy or 2- 3 days after chemotherapy
c) At the time of nausea, during chemotherapy
d) One week before or after chemotherapy

Question 214: Before Administering with cyclophosphamide, which among the following medication from the patient's drug profile has to be reported?
a) Celexa
b) Allopurinol
c) Elavil
d) Amoxicillin

Question 215: What will be the advice of the nurse, when a 64 year old African American patient asks about the prostate screening for her grown sons?

a) An ultrasound guided biopsy of the prostate ate the beginning of age 45

b) A MRI scan at the age of 45

c)A prostate specific antigen test at the age of 45

d) Sulphonyl acid phosphatase at the age of 45

Question 216: A patient's temperature is 39*C and she has tachypnea, tachycardia and leukocytosis (20,000/mm3).She is an immunocompromised patient and she has developed a systematic infection. The infection would be classified as:

a) Multi organ disinfection syndrome

b) Systemic inflammatory response syndrome.

c) Bacteremia.

d) None of the above.

Question 217: A patient with permanent colostomy expresses concern of having sexual intercourse. What will the nurse recommend initially?

a) Replace ostomy appliance just before the sexual intercourse

b) Have food before engaging in sexual intercourse

c) Track bowel habits to schedule sexual intercourse

d) Discuss with the therapist before having a sexual intercourse

Question 218: A patient who is undergoing treatment has to be more concerned about intimacy. Which among the following is said to be the most appropriate intervention while discussing this with the patient?

a) Using PLISSIT model to promote discussion

b) Limiting the discussion to reduce further discomfort

c) Referring all further discussion to the physician

d) Telling the patient to focus only on treatment

Question 219: Adjuvant chemotherapy is recommended after undergoing surgery for cancer. Here adjuvant chemotherapy is referred to?

a) Immunotherapy are used to boost body's immune system

b) Drug given to target minimal disease or metastasis

c) Proper investigation of the drugs used along with surgery

d) Treatment are given to the patient who cannot tolerate pain

Question 220: Within a week of chemotherapy a patient with acute lymphoid leukemia experience the following symptoms; Hyperkalemia, Hyperphosphatemia and Hypocalcemia. The above symptoms indicate?

a) Hyponatremia and hypo-osmolality

b) Septic shock

c) Tumor Lysis Syndrome

d) Consumptive coagulopathy

Question 221: Despite the use of antiemetics, Megan reports of nausea and vomiting before every chemotherapy. She starts crying and requests to stop the treatment. How will the nurse calms down Megan?

a) By explaining that everyone experience nausea and Vomiting

b) By suggesting the healthcare provider to stop treatment

c) By discussing integrative therapy options

d) By recommending healthcare provider to reduce dosage

Question 222: Watson experiences his anger about the diagnosis of cancer as he was about to receive his first chemotherapy. What would be response given by the nurse?

a) Suggest Watson to participate in treatment plan

b) Asks the physician to delay the treatment

c) Suggest way for the patient to participate in the treatment plan

d) Initiating a referral to social worker

Question 223: William who has lung cancer reports of the following symptoms; A sudden acute pleura pain on his left side. He also exhibits dyspnea, Tachypnea, tachycardia, slight cough, and decreased sound in breathing over his left chest. These symptoms are due to?

a) Myocardial infarction

b) Lymphoma

c) Pneumothorax on left side

d) Acute chest pain

Question 224: The primary purpose of providing multidisciplinary oncology care is to?

a) Meet the regulatory standards

b) Deliver cost effective services

c) Improvise patient's communication

d) Improve patient's outcome

Question 225: Which among the following is considered as a true positive indication from cancer screening?

a) The individual has cancer

b) The individual has a symptom for future diagnosis of cancer

c) The patient doesn't have cancer despite of positive result

d) The patient has cancer despite of the negative result

Question 226: Aching and throbbing at a particular region is described as?

a) Neuropathic pain

b) Pain in the internal organ

c) Somatic pain

d) Referred pain

Question 227: Which of the following action exemplifies safe practice for Robin who has an implanted intrathecal cup for pain management?

a) Arrangements for Robin to have the pump refilling for every 7 months
b) Cleansing the lock port with sanitizer before each use
c) Tracing the path of tube from the patient to pump
d) Special tubes with injection ports

Question 228: Watson expresses his willingness to return back to work after treatment. But sometimes he reports of feeling fatigue. Which among the following is considered as the suitable step for his problem?

a) Discussing with his officials regarding flexible work time.
b) Avoiding discussion with his co-workers who are sick
c) Having a break for a 2 years before commencing work schedule
d) Asking the family member to work and continue with household chores.

Question 229: Clara, a 20 year old childhood brain cancer survivor is complaining about her sudden weight gain, weakness in muscles, dysmenorrhea and depression. At the age of 5, she underwent radiation therapy and surgery as treatment for cancer. The above symptoms are the later effects of?

a) Resurgence of Cancer
b) Cardiomyopathy
c) Lack of healthy red blood cells
d) Hypothyroidism

Question 230: What is reason for administering whole breast radiation following Lumpectomy for a patient with stage 1 breast cancer?

a) To remove microscopic disease
b) To remove nodal disease
c) To reduce communicable disease
d) To decrease locally advanced disease

Question 231: What will be the most appropriate test that the nurse suggest when Ricard's adolescent son approaches for screening?

a) Colonoscopy

b) CA 19-9 test

c) Prostate-specific antigen test

d) Testicular self-examination

Question 232: Merlin is a foreign born women with breast cancer. She has a lower survival rate when compared to other women with breast cancer who were born in the United States. Which among the following is more likely to attribute to Merlin's condition?

a) Histologic grades of the tumor

b) Differences in the protocol of treatment

c) Access to mammographic treatment

d) Country from where the women have been immigrated.

Question 233: The most prominent symptom of oral mucositis is?

a) Bleeding

b) Eye Infection

c) Pain

d) Headache

Question 234: A patient with breast cancer reports of exhaustion after 3 months of chemotherapy and radiation. How will the nurse respond?

a) Explains the importance of sleep

b) " Physician will suggest antidepressants"

c) Explains that the side effects shall reduce very soon

d) Asks the patient to express the ways it affects the daily routine

Question 235: Focus is made on palliative care for the patient and family in order to:

a) Treat every patient equally in order to meet his / her needs, expectations and cultural beliefs

b) Attend the need of those who love and care for the dying person

c) Provide relief from suffering during the last 6 months of life expectancy

d) Preserve the patient life that is based solely on Clinical technology and scientific advances

Question 236: During her childhood, Rosie has received Carmustine. Now, being a 24 year old adult she reports of persistent cough and shortness in breath. Which of the following has high risk of development?

a) Lung embolism

b) Pulmonary Fibrosis

c) Accumulation of pus in pleural space

d) Allergic reaction to the fungus

Question 237: Juliette has stage III C ovarian cancer. After receiving her first line therapy, she became worst again after a little improvement. She demonstrates an understanding of her condition by stating that,

a) " I think I must be overdoing it a bit"

b) " These symptoms are due to chemotherapy"

c)" I'm happy that I won't be needing any additional treatment"

d) " Are clinical trials available for other recurrent disease?"

Question 238: While developing cancer therapies, it is important to have an understanding about the immunology because:

a) It shows how free radicals are removed from the body

b) It identifies how T cells, B cells and natural killer cells work

c) It assumes the duration of treatment tolerance

d) It creates an impact on treatment choices to maintain the bone marrow function

Question 239: An 85 years old patient was advised for a surgery and chemotherapy by his physician. But his family members were not convinced with the physician's decision.

They advocate palliative care. What will be the response from the nurse when asked by the patient?
a) Assess the patient's values and basis for his preference.
b) Consults hospital ethics committee
c) Helps the patient in completing advanced directives
d) Supports and documents family's preference

Question 240: How does the alkylating agent exert their pressure?
a) By disrupting folate dependent metabolic process essential for cell replication
b) By attaching to CD52 on the surface of B and T cells that generally result in antibody dependent lysis.
c) By binding to the DNA strand which prevents DNA replication and cell division
d) By causing the release of toxic free radicals inside the cell and triggering their apoptosis.

Question 241: Which of the following has to be administered as initial treatment for the patient with septic shock?
a) IV antifungals
b) Corticosteroids at high dosage
c) IV antibiotics
d) Vasopressors

Question 242: A cancer survivor is applying for a job interview. Which among the following should be done by the applicant during the initial interview?
a) The applicant has to explain about the personal qualifications for the job
b) The applicant has to provide medical information and current status
c) The applicant has to contact the interviewer
d) The applicant should not provide details about his cancer treatment

Question 243: Michelle has metastatic breast cancer. She experiences pain at the site of

metastasis during the initiation of tamoxifen. Which among the following clearly explains the pain?

a) Due to progression of disease

b) Due to improper sleeping position

c) A Psychosomatic reaction due to the diagnosis of metastasis

d) A common temporary reaction to the initiation therapy

Question 244: To whom is the nurse responsible to according to ANA code of ethics?

a) Physician

b) Medical Council

c) Patient

d) Herself

Question 245: A patient named Michael Smith is seen shaking and distraught when the nurse enters his room. Michael has just spoken with his doctor. After seeing the patient's condition the nurse's response should be:

a) Everything will be alright, don't worry.

b) Can I get something for you?

c) Shall I contact your family?

d) You seem worried and shaken, are you alright?

Question 246: Which of the following intervention is suggested to the patient who has dry desquamation?

a) Hydrogel dressing

b) Aloe Vera dressing

c) Moisturizing skin cream

d) Silver sulphadiazine

Question 247: Why is it important to assess attitudes about illness and care-seeking in a patient from different racial and ethnic groups?

a) To determine ineffective intervention

b) Tailor treatment approaches to individual patient

c) To effectively change attitudes.

d) To identify socio economic status of the patient.

Question 248: The work of epidermal growth factor receptor inhibitors inside the cell is to
a) Block the binding on the intracellular portion of the receptor
b) Promote the proliferation of non-malignant cells to repair
c) Produce antibodies in recognizing and destroying cancer cells
d) Activate the T cells to mount an immune system attack on cancer cells

Question 249: Regina's pain was under control after administering morphine sulfate but due to other side effects she was administered with equianalgesic drug. At what range should the dosage of new drug be initiated?
a) 25- 50% below equianalgesic drug
b) 25- 50% above the equianalgesic drug
c) 5% below equianalgesic drug
d) 20% above equianalgesic drug

Question 250: Robert has pulmonary metastasis and has been receiving repeated thoracentesis. Which among the following development will the nurse be more concerned about?
a) lung expansion minimization (trapped lung)
b) Lung embolism
c) Constriction of airways in the lung
d) Pneumonitis

Question 251: A cancer patient reports of following symptoms; appearance of white lesions on the tongue and inside of her cheeks, the tissues is irritated painful with slight bleeding. Which among the following is the best treatment?
a) Ampicillin

b) Caphosol

c) Mouth wash with lemon swabs

d) Nystatin an antifungal medication for oral suppression

Question 252: A patient is treated with posaconazole. Which of the following side effects should be informed to the patient regarding the treatment?

a) Pancreatitis

b) Torsades de Pointes

c) Anemia

d) Bone marrow aplasia

Question 253: The formal closure activities that should be done once the patient dies are:

a) Helping the family in making funeral rituals.

b) Establishing an ongoing long relationship.

c) Sending a condolence card.

d) All of the above.

Question 254: Rochelle has been diagnosed with breast cancer and she is 14 weeks pregnant. She is more concerned about the treatment effects on her baby. Which among the following information does the nurse provide?

a) Occurrence of spontaneous abortion

b) Decrease in doses to ensure safety

c) About the initiation of chemotherapy after pregnancy

d) Minimal effects of chemotherapy after first trimester

Question 255: When developing an education program which of the following action must be performed first?

a) Determine educational objective

b) Formulating criteria for evaluation

c) Assess learning needs

d) Educational methods had to be selected

Question 256: Which of the following terminology is associated with the malignant tumor originating in the epithelial cells?

a) Adeno and squamous
b) Osteo and Condra
c) Lympho and Myelo
d) Lipo and Condra

Question 257: Which among the following is an example for adaptive or specific immunity?

a) Large lymphocyte production
b) Cell mediated response
c) Inflammatory response
d) Acute phase protein production

Question 258: A patient has a platelet count of 15000/ mm³. Which of following intervention should the nurse institute while attending the patient?

a) Providing massage to reduce the pain
b) Placing warm hot bags on the injected region
c) Using mouth swabs to complete oral care
d) Obtaining blood samples through large needles

Question 259: Richard reports of certain symptoms after receiving a high dose of external beam radiation for lung cancer 8 weeks ago. This symptoms include development of dyspnea and non productive cough. In the area of his previous radiation treatment, a chest x-ray shows open ground glass opacification. Which among the following is the result of the above symptoms?

a) Radiation pneumonitis
b) Increased libidos
c) Bilateral atelectasis
d) Cardiac tamponade

Question 260: A nurse has been assigned to take care of 5 patients. She provides documentation and assessment for only 4 patients as she had misread the entire agreement. The legal principle that applies to this situation is?

a) Non harming
b) Breach of duty
c) Dereliction of duty
d) Testimonial proof

Question 261: Among the following, the early symptoms for increased intracranial pressure is related to?

a) Confusion
b) Nausea
c) Fatigue
d) Decortication

Question 262: Bob is said to have frequent seizure despite of receiving hospice service for brain tumor. He was not able tolerate oral Anticonvulsants as he has only limited days for survival. What will be the nurse's anticipation?

a) Keppra
b) Liquid lorazepam
c) Fentanyl patch
d) Phenothiazine

Question 263: Which of the following medications requires mandatory enrollment in a program to ensure teaching about risks to a fetus is provided?

a) Capecitabine
b) Sorafenib
c) Lenalidomide
d) Everolimus

Question 264: What is the long term complication for the patient who is receiving hormonal therapy for prostate cancer?

a) Cardiac dysfunction

b) Lymphedema

c) Adverse skeletal events

d) Ulcers

Question 265: Merlin, a cancer patient has lost four pounds since the beginning of her Chemotherapy-treatment. What will be first reaction of the nurse after finding it during her home visit?

a) Asks Merlin to consult physician

b) Suggests high-protein and high calorie-food

c) Investigates the reason for weight loss

d) Arrange for meals on the wheels service

Question 266: Robin has been diagnosed with lung cancer and admitted in the hospital. He will be discharged after he gets administered with cisplatin and etoposide. What are the information that are included in the discharge report?

a) Careful observation of urine for the next two days for blood and immediately report its presence.

b) Development of hiccups are considered as normal

c) A fever should be reported immediately to the physician

d) Ringing in the ear continues to increase due to etoposide

Question 267: William was diagnosed with acute myeloid leukemia. He reported of bleeding gums and refracts to random donor platelets. Which among the following has to be anticipated initially?

a) Obtaining a type and crosshatching for cryoprecipitate

b) CMV-negative platelets can be transfused

c) Administer human leukocyte antigen-matched platelets

d) Fresh frozen plasma can be administered

Question 268: Richard has completed treatment for neck and head cancer. He is at high risk for which secondary malignancy?

a) Kidney cancer

b) Bile duct cancer

c) Lung cancer

d) Glioblastoma multiforme

Question 269: Patient who has been undergoing treatment for cancer fails to respond to the treatment. When this has been informed to the patient, what will be the initial nursing interventions?

a) Asks the patient to share the feelings after hearing the news

b) Providing time for self processing by the patient

c) Asking family members to provide verbal support

d) Reviewing the treatment possibilities as referred by the physician

Question 270: From which among the following does the squamous cell carcinoma of esophagus tends to arise?

a) Abdominal esophagus

b) Proximal esophagus

c) Lymph

d) Hyaline cartilage

Question 271: There is a significant increase in the risk of developing a breast cancer. Which among the following people has a higher chance of risk?

a) Menarche at age 13

b) First pregnancy at age of 31

c) Mother diagnosed before 60 years of age

d) Menopause at the age of 53

Question 272: Pathological process of syndrome of inappropriate anti-diuretic hormone include?

a) Decreased sodium secretion by kidneys.

b) Urine osmolality is less than serum osmolality

c) Increased serum sodium concentration

d) Increased reabsorption of water by the renal tubules

Question 273: **Which of the following side effects has an increased risk for the patient who is receiving Bevacizumab exhibiting proteinuria?**

a) Mucositis

b) Cardiac dysfunction

c) Hypertension

d) Peripheral neuropathy

Question 274: **Clara is a premenopausal patient who has been diagnosed with cancer. After the treatment, when can Clara expect her menstruation again?**

a) After 6 months

b) After 3 months

c) After 2 years

d) After a year

Question 275: **How does filgrastim maintains the dose intensity of the treatment regimen?**

a) By reducing the risk of damaging the heart muscle

b) By reducing the occurrence of Nausea

c) By reducing the febrile neutropenia occurrence

d) By saving the body from the attack of toxic substance (Leucovorin rescue).

Question 276: **William, a cancer patient plans of going through a clinical trial that compares current standard treatment with a chemotherapeutic agent. Which among the following denotes the exact phase of this trial?**

a) 5

b) 7

c) 3

d) 2

Question 277: Among the following, who has increased risk of developing a graft-versus-host disease?
a) A 30-years- old patient received an autologous hematopoietic stem cells transfer
b) A 60-years-old patient received an allogeneic transplant from a unrelated donor.
c) A 25-years-old patient received a tandem autologous stem cell transplant
d) A 42-years- old patient received a syngeneic hematopoietic stem cell transplant

Question 278: Michael, a 25 year old patient has been diagnosed with cancer. Physician prescribed him with temozolomide. What will be the initial instruction given to the patient?
a) Medication must be taken at bedtime on an empty stomach
b) Ingestion of medicine with full glass of milk
c) Medication must be taken after dinner
d) Always consume a magnesium supplement

Question 279: After hematopoietic stem cell transplant, Robert was taught about the discharge medication. Which among the following explains the purpose of tacrolimus?
a) It helps to prevent fungal pneumonia
b) It avoids sinusoidal obstruction syndrome
c) It prevents graft-versus-host disease
d) It prevents Nausea and vomiting sensation

Question 280: David is 70 year old having prostate cancer and vertebral tenderness . He bears so much pain during his bowel movements. He also suffering with muscle loss and sensory paresthesia. The appropriate cause for this is:
a) urinary infection
b) spinal cord compression
c) Lower Back strain
d) loss of urine or bowel control

Question 281: Which of the following has the possibility to occur as secondary malignancy for Rochelle who has ovarian cancer?

a) Hodgkin carcinoma

b) Ocular Melanoma

c) Leiomyosarcoma

d) Gastric carcinoma

Question 282: Among the following, which is termed as the shortest phase of the cell cycle?

a) Meiosis

b) Prophase

c) Gap 1

d) Mitosis

Question 283: Which among the following statements indicate the need for additional teaching regarding the coverage provided by the Family Medical Leave Act?

a) " I know I'm eligible because I'm an American citizen"

b) " I can take up to 15 weeks of leave "

c)" It helps me to take good care of my sister who is also a cancer patient "

d) " It is difficult because my time off is unpaid "

Question 284: A patient is suddenly diagnosed with surgical unresectable renal cell carcinoma that has suddenly metastasized to Liver. Which of the following biological therapy has to be prescribed?

a) Intravenous drug temsirolimus

b) Adrucil (flurouracil)

c) epidermal growth factor receptor (EGFR) inhibitor (Cetuximab)

d) Nilotinib

Question 285: Which among the following technique supports the healthy communication pattern between the patient and nurse?

a) After providing all the information, the questions has to be limited.

b) The objective and factual information has to be provided regarding the treatment plan

c) Physical distance has to be established between the parties

d) Feedbacks has to be obtained regarding the preferences and experiences

Question 286: A patient after first chemotherapy experiences chemotherapy induced alopecia. Which among the following indicates the time frame of alopecia?

a) After 1 month

b) After 2 month

c) Before 24 hours

d) After 2 weeks

Question 287: Which of the following cancer is associated with a patient exposed to radon for a longer duration?

a) Bladder Cancer

b) Colorectal / Bowel Cancer

c) Lung Cancer

d) Breast Cancer

Question 288: In order to reduce the noise rattled breathing for a dying patient which of the following non pharmacological interventions is suitable?

a) Humidifying oxygen

b) Executing nasopharyngeal suctions

c) Increasing the morphine infusion rate

d) Relocating/Repositioning to clear secretion

Question 289: The highest incident and mortality of prostate is reported among which of the following groups in United States of America?

a) Hispanic Americans

b) Asian Americans

c) Non Hispanic Caucasian

d) African Americans

Question 290: Which among the following measures provides relief for the patient who has had persistent nausea and vomiting despite of receiving medication for controlling the symptoms?

a) By laying flat on the floor

b) By avoiding dinner

c) By taking a deep breath and having control of swallowing manners

d) By in taking large volume of fluid

Question 291: A common and preventable cause of anxiety in Robin who is suffering from cancer is?

a) Disturbances in sleep

b) Uncontrolled pain

c) Changes in the treatment protocol

d) Spiritual distress

Question 292: While getting Doxorubicin infused Mike reports Pruritus above the peripheral IV site. The nurse observes a redness along the vein with a brisk sustained blood return. Which among the following reactions does the above symptoms indicate?

a) An Extravasation

b) Flare reaction

c) Radiation recall

d) Psychosomatic response

Question 293: Occurrence of nausea is generally due to cancer or due to the treatment of cancer. Patient are taught with some basic self-care strategies that encourages patients to ?

a) Eat food that are cold at room temperature

b) High protein and potassium rich food

c) Avoid brushing after nauseating

d) Consume sauces and gravies

Question 294: Clara has been diagnosed with stage 3 cervical cancer. There are certain situations in which she may defer discussions about alteration in body image and sexual intimacy prior to the cancer treatment. Which among the following is likely to match the above reasons?

a) Depersonalization of the disease experience

b) Expectations of unrealistic outcomes

c) Concerned of being perceived as vain.

d) Expectation of experiencing minimal symptom for treatment

Question 295: What is duration within which manifestation of the symptoms for anaphylactic reaction occur?

a) 60 minutes

b) 45 minutes

c) 30 minutes

d) 20 minutes

Question 296: The protective equipment that is recommended during the clean-up of the hazardous medical spill is

a) Cloth gown

b) Face shield

c) Vinyl surgical gloves

d) Latex gloves

Question 297: A patient with renal carcinoma has been administered with sunitinib. Patient reports of burning sensation, tingling and redness in the palm and foot while receiving sunitinib. Which among the following is the result of the above symptoms?

a) Acneiform rash

b) Erythema multiform major

c) Darkened patches and spots on skin

d) Palmar plantar erythrodysesthesia

Question 298: William has been newly diagnosed with Hodgkin lymphoma. Through the following clinical diagnosis, William is determined to have an unfavorable prognosis?

a) Involvement of several lymph nodes
b) Absolute lymphocyte count 400/ mm³
c) Hemoglobin 15g/dl
d) Thrombocytopenia

Question 299: The required premedication causes drowsiness. The nurse informs the patient about the drowsiness that occurs due to medication. Therefore the patient request the nurse for delaying the treatment so that patient performs the prayer during sunset. The nurse should first

a) Require that a waiver be signed to delay treatment
b) Delay the treatment for 24 hours
c) Assess to determine if a delay is permissible
d) Informing the patient that the treatment can't be delayed

Question 300: William reports difficulty in manipulating a toothbrush and silverware before administering fourth dose of cisplatin. Which among the following is said to be the initial intervention?

a) Arranging an occupational therapy consultation.
b) Document the findings and reporting to the physician
c) Instructing the patient to take seek attention regarding meals and oral hygiene
d) Assuring patient that these are temporary side effects of chemotherapy

Question 301. A 41-year-old women is diagnosed to be suffering from stage IV ovarian cancer. She requests to consult a different doctor because she believes that her doctor has misdiagnosed her. Which stage of Elizabeth Kubler-Ross's stages of grief is she currently suffering from?

a) Denial

b) Bargaining
c) Anger
d) Betrayal

Answer Key with explanation for 300 Question

Question 1: The complications that occur after performing percutaneous lung biopsy is?

a) Pneumonia

b) Pneumothorax

c) Acute or partial collapse of lung or section of lung

d) Building up of fluid between the lung and tissues (Pleural effusion)

Answer: b

Explanation: Insertion of spinal type of needle into the chest cavity for obtaining tissue for examination is known as Lung biopsy. Generally air gets introduced into the lung region causing pneumothorax.

Question 2: For managing nausea and Vomiting at the end of the life, which of the following complimentary is most likely to be effective?

a) Walking

b) Massage

c) Acupuncture

d) Music therapy

Answer: d

Explanation: Music therapy can be used for facilitating movement and overall physical rehabilitation and motivating clients to cope with treatment. It tends to reduce the duration of nausea and vomiting.

Question 3: A patient with lymphoma feels weak while ambulating and dribbling urine and also experience numbness in feet. Which among the following will be the initial suspect by the nurse?

a) Peripheral neuritis

b) Endocrine disruptor

c) Type 1 diabetes

d) Spinal cord compression

Answer: d

Explanation: Lymphatic cancer is a risk to spinal cord compression that includes weakness in leg, loss of sensation and loss of urine or bowel control.

Question 4: Advantage of implanted vascular system over a tunneled central vascular system is?

a) Low cost of insertion

b) Reduced risk of infection

c) Short term usage

d) Unlimited ability to access

Answer: b

Explanation: One main advantage of implanted ports over tunneled central venous catheters is the reduced risk of infection.

Question 5: A patient is at the dying stage due to lung cancer. The patient also feels dyspneic. What will the nurse do to make the patient feel less short of breath after finding that his bed is elevated to 45° and also noticed that he is receiving oxygen at 4L / min?

a) The nurse will make the patient lie flat on bed

b) The nurse will turn the airflow of the pedestal fan towards the patient

c) The nurse tries to have a conversation with the patient

d) The nurse informs this to a physician

Answer: b

Explanation: By directing the fan towards the patient, the patient shall overcome the fear of feeling short of breath. By making the patient lie flat on bed doesn't increase the airflow. Usually 2 to 4L/ min oxygen is administered to the patient. By altering the fluid intake does not affect dyspnea as the breathlessness is associated with lung cancer.

Question 6: In order to prevent the occurrence of colon cancer, which among the following plays a major role?
 a) Daily exercise
 b) Diet planning
 c) Acetaminophen
 d) Vitamins
Answer: b
Explanation: Researches prove that occurrence of colon cancer can be prevented by maintaining proper diet plans. This reduces the chance of occurrence from 60 to 80%.

Question 7: What happens when Mathew gets infused with cryopreserved hematopoietic stem cells?
 a) The preservative shall cause a garlic-like taste and odor.
 b) This cell infusion happens in a period of 4 days
 c) Urine will be pink-tinged at least for a week after infusion
 d) IN order to observe the changes, premedication shall not be administered
Answer: a
Explanation: Hematopoietic stem cells have been used for the treatment of both hematological and non-hematological disease; while more recently mesenchymal stem cells derived from bone marrow have been the subject of both laboratory and early clinical studies DMSO is known to be toxic to tissues and cells, with toxicity being time, temperature and concentration dependent. When Mathew gets infused with cryopreserved Hematopoietic cells, DMSO causes garlic- like taste and odor.

Question 8: A nurse is working with a patient with terminal illness. Which among the following statement seems to be helpful for her in assisting her patient to reframe hope?
 a) "We are always there to help you"
 b) "You are still left with more time, don't worry"

c) "Have faith in God, he will save you"

d) "What appears to be more important to you?"

Answer: d

Explanation: By asking the patient about his or her importance can make the patient to focus on the goals while reframing hope. While some patients want to spend time with their family or complete any incomplete task while other patient will find this as a pain free. The nurse must help the patient along with the healthcare member to identify the patient's goal and should make sure that plans are made to make the patient achieve his or her goal.

Question 9: A patient continues to work full time even after being fatigue due to radiation therapy. Which will be the most useful suggestion among the following?

a) Start working earlier and complete before the energy   levels drop.

b) Keep all the frequently used items under close reach

c) Engage in aerobics workout for 2 hours

d) Involve muscular activity during the worktime

Answer: b

Explanation: Fatigue occurs when the patient is about to drain all the energy. It is advisable to reduce manual work by keeping the required things within reach and avoid fastening that reduces the stamina.

Question 10: At what age prostate specific antigen blood test has to be taken in order to reduce average risk according to American Cancer society Guidelines?

a) 50

b) 20

c) 30

d) 40

Answer: a

Explanation: According to the American Cancer Society Guidelines, in order to avoid average risk of prostate cancer in men, prostate specific antigen blood test has to be taken at the age of 50.

Question 11: William is experiencing uncontrolled pain due to bone metastasis. The nurse, the patient and the palliative care are reviewing the plan of care. The above scenario is an example of?

a) Advising

b) Criticize

c) Collaboration

d) Advising

Answer: c

Explanation: In order to plan efficiently for pain management, the oncology nurse and other members of the palliative care are advised to work along with the patient and their family.

Question 12: Clara returns home to take care of her mother who becomes terminally ill. Her father disagrees with her mother's choice regarding terminal care whereas Clara agrees with her father's choice. They try convincing her mother by applying pressure. This is an example of which theory according to Bowen's Family system?

a) Sentimental

b) Triangular theory

c) Transition

d) Evolution

Answer: b

Explanation: This situation appears as an example for Triangular theory. This theory states that two persons are considered basic individual but when the problem arises ,the involvement of a third person is brought between the stable unit. According to the Bowen's family system, two people supporting and one person opposing occurs as a common result. This theory suggest that individual should look up on the issue depending upon his or her family members as the change in one person's behavior can affect other members in the family.

Question 13: Which of the following below requires immediate assessments?

a) Velcade under the skin

b) Vincristine administered reaches cerebrospinal fluid

c) Asparaginase is given into large muscles

d) Intra peritoneal cisplatin

Answer: b

Explanation: Intrathecal administer of vincristine is fatal

Question 14: To identify, monitor and improve the effectiveness of oncology nursing care, nurse has collected the data and analyzed it. The above nursing practice exemplifies the?

 a) Patient's advocacy standards

 b) Collaboration standard

 c) Resource utilization standards

 d) Collegiality standards

Answer: c

Explanation: Resource utilization is a metric that shows whether your whole team or specific employees are fully booked. In order to maximize the patient's outcomes, resource utilization requires the nurse to evaluate, criticize and mobilize the most appropriate resources.

Question 15: Richardson, a 69 year old patient report of sudden increase in temperature of 101°F (38.3°c) and lightheadedness, he received his Chemotherapy a week ago. The nurse identifies that Richard must be dyspneic and diaphoretic. What will be the nurse initial response?

 a) Recheck temperature in 2 hours

 b) Report to emergency department

 c) Call for an ambulance

 d) Take paracetamol

Answer: c

Explanation: The time at which chemotherapy exerts its maximum effect on the bone marrow and the white blood count reaches its lowest point is the worst moment of the situation. This usually occurs within 7 to 10 days after administration. Patients are most susceptible to infections at this time due to neutropenia (low count of white blood cells). Patients over 65 years are at greater risk and if they are untreated this causes shock and results in death.

Question 16: Persistent fever and chills has been reported by a patient receiving interleukin 2 with neutrophils count of 1500/mm³. What is the representation of these symptoms?

 a) Tumor lysis syndrome

 b) Septic shock

 c) Drug induced reaction

 d) Viral infection

Answer: c

Explanation: Stimulation is based generally on host cytotoxic and immunological response. Therefore the most common side effect will be the flu like symptoms.

Question 17: **What will be the choice of treatment for the patient with stage 1 non-small cell lung cancer with impaired pulmonary functions?**
a) Removal of lobe of an organ (lobectomy)
b) Removal of Lung (pneumactomy)
c) External beam radiation
d) Platinum based chemotherapy

Answer: c

Explanation: Radiation therapy are received by non-surgical candidates due to impaired lung Function. This is generally curative for the patients with stage 1 and 2 cancer.

Question 18: **What is the additional role of corticosteroids along with decreasing inflammation?**
a) Reduce anxiety
b) Improves muscle tone
c) Stimulate the appetite
d) Stimulate weight loss

Answer: c

Explanation: Dexamethasone and Prednisone are some of the corticosteroids that stimulate appetite that can create a sense of well-being with increase in weight.

Question 19: **Tiara is said to receive her fourth dose of chemotherapy for lung cancer. She experiences nausea suddenly while driving to hospital for her treatment. Which among the following is the type of nausea that Tiara experiences?**
a) Overcoming or Breakthrough
b) Delayed
c) Anticipatory
d) Acute

Answer: c

Explanation: Patterns of nausea and vomiting ranges in etiology and duration. Acute nausea and vomiting generally occurs within several minutes to several hours after the drug is being administered. Delayed nausea and vomiting develops after or more than 24 hours of drug administration. Breakthrough nausea and vomiting occurs when the preventative regimens fail. Anticipatory nausea and vomiting is a conditioned response that occurs prior to the administration of chemotherapy.

Question 20: **Swelling in the left arm and fingers are reported by patient who underwent mastectomy 3 days ago. While vascular access device is easily flushed, blood return is not obtained. Which case will be suspected among the following?**
a) Thrombosis within the superior Vena Cava
b) Delayed anaphylactic reaction to paclitaxel
c) Prolonged dependency of arm positioning
d) Lymphedema after mastectomy
Answer: a
Explanation: Thrombosis should be considered as the central venous access device can be generally flushed but blood return can't be expected upon aspiration.

Question 21: **When is adjuvant therapy administered in the case of Breast Cancer?**
a) While locally treating cancer cells with minimal harm to other cells
b) It doesn't require specific time to be administered and can cure the patient by killing the cancer cells
c) After the primary therapy in order to increase the chance of disease free survival for a long term.
d) Before primary therapy, to shrink the tumor that is in operable in its current state
Answer: c
Explanation: The major role of adjuvant therapy is to target the minimal residual disease for the patients who are at the risk of developing metastasis.

Question 22: **Which among the following is said to be the most distressing side effects for the patients undergoing chemotherapy, radiotherapy or biotherapy?**
a) Nausea
b) Breathlessness
c) Vomiting
d) Fatigue
Answer: d
Explanation: The most distressing side effect for the patient undergoing chemotherapy,

radiotherapy and biotherapy is fatigue. It means of tiredness with low energy and a strong desire to sleep.

Question 23: What type of nausea does the patient receive after 48 hours of chemotherapy?
 a) Somatic
 b) Delayed
 c) Short term
 d) Breakthrough
Answer: b
Explanation: Despite progress in treating chemotherapy-induced nausea and vomiting (CINV), especially in the acute phase up to 24 hours after treatment, the condition is still one of the side effects in patient and delays in getting cured.

Question 24: Mortality rate can be reduced by using acetyl salicylic acid for which of the following cancer types?
 a) Gastrointestinal
 b) Malignant neoplasm of testis
 c) Cervical
 d) Leukemia
Answer: a
Explanation: Acetyl salicylic acid also known as aspirin generally reduces people's risk on cancer by frequent use. It is also said to reduce the mortality rate of gastrointestinal cancer.

Question 25: Which of the following actions characterize the social learning theory?
 a) Collaborating to solve problems
 b) Trying to goals
 c) Trying to imitate other's activity
 d) Creating mnemonics
Answer: c
Explanation: Learning usually takes place only by watching and imitating others activities according to the social learning theory.

Question 26: The policy and procedure for chemotherapy administration has been reviewed by nurse's manager. In what ways can the ASCO/ ONS Chemotherapy Administration for Safety Standards assist in this process?

a) It provides idea about the professional responsibility of the oncology nurses in chemotherapy administration.

b) It helps in providing description for the oncology nurse jobs

c) The required educational classes for the oncology nurses are being listed

d) The data collection tool regarding the quality improvement are provided

Answer: a

Explanation: The ASCO/ OND ensures the safety standards for the administration of chemotherapy. This generally conveys the staffing issue, chemotherapy planning preparation and administration.

Question 27: What is considered as the most important factor for self-determined closure of life?

a) Honoring wishes of patient regarding end of life care

b) Discharging the patient

c) Stopping the treatment

d) Proceeding with advanced medication

Answer: a

Explanation: The best way is to honor the patient's wish regarding the end of life care. In some cases, family members decide the patient's wish regardless of the patient's individual wish. And in other cases patients are unable to make any decisions. During these cases the health care providers and care givers are more aware of the patient's wish and therefore ensure that the patient's wish is honored.

Question 28: Clara has a history of ovarian cancer suddenly reports feeling full after eating small quantity and also experiences an increase in weight. She has noticed an increase of 10 pounds within a week and also states that she is eating less. What will the nurse instruct Clara?

a) Eat small and frequent meals

b) Visit the clinic

c) Report if there is an increase in weight

d) Call when is there is an increase in swelling of ankle.

Answer: b

Explanation: Bowel obstruction incident has been reported between 5.5% and 42% of patients with ovarian cancer. Symptoms include vomiting, distention, colicky pain, and diarrhea. However, signs of bowel movements depend on the location of obstruction. Medical treatment includes relieving the distention, correcting the fluid imbalances, and removing the source of the obstruction.

Question 29: Paclitaxel (PTX), sold under the brand name Taxol among others, is a chemotherapy medication used to treat a number of types of cancer. Harry is administered with the first dose of PTX. He will undergo certain reactions. For which among the following, the nurse should have made the arrangements to treat the Harry?
 a) Hypersensitivity reaction
 b) Feeling of being in a cold environment with shivering and chills
 c) Urinary Retention
 d) Vomiting
Answer: a
Explanation: Hypersensitivity is the side effects associated with Harry. Hypersensitivity can be localized or systemic with exaggerated or inappropriate immune response. Some other effects include increased sweating, nausea, dry mouth. Administering with cimetidine, diphenhydramine as a pretreatment process can prevent hypersensitivity.

Question 30: Which among the following clearly denotes the 'purpose of a living will' ,as taught by the nurse?
 a) Appointing surrogate to make medical decisions
 b) Making final decision regarding treatment progression
 c) Establishment of the patient's desire for care prior to a life threatening illness
 d) Acknowledgement of the risk and limiting the recommended therapies
Answer: c
Explanation: In case of any terminal illness, the determination of care that a patient is willing to receive is based on the patient's willingness to live.

Question 31: Katie with family history of BRCA1 and BRCA2 breast cancer is 20 years old. She enquires about the initiating mammogram. What will the nurse recommend?
 a) Having an early mammogram at the age of 35 years
 b) Having a breast ultrasound after her first pregnancy

c) Talking with her doctor about advantages and disadvantages of starting the screening earlier.

d) To begin her screening exactly when her family was identified.

Answer: c

Explanation: Mammograms are advised every year after the age of 40. But women with increased risk due to family history are advised to have a conversation with the doctor regarding the effects of early mammogram.

Question 32: Mathew complains of itching at the infusion site while administering doxorubicin peripherally. The nurse's initial response to the red streak along with the blood return will be?

 a) Continue the drug administration

 b) Stop the infusion and flush the line with saline

 c) Change the IV site

 d) Stop the infusion and instill the antidote

Answer: b

Explanation: A local venous inflammatory response with subsequent histamine release manifested by streaking or red blotches along the vein without pain is termed as flare reaction. If the extravasation of drug is stopped, then the infusion should also stop and the line should be flushed with saline while watching for the flare resolution.

Question 33: In order to reduce anxiety which among the following is suggested?

 a) Hyperbaric oxygen therapy

 b) Allopathy

 c) Meditation

 d) Mindfulness-based stress reduction

Answer: d

Explanation: Anxiety disorders include panic attacks, obsessive-compulsive disorder and post-traumatic stress disorder. This can be reduced by mindfulness based stress reduction therapy.

Question 34: Certain medication can cause increased sedation when administered with opioids. Which of the following medication is the correct option?

 a) Narcan

 b) Glutocorticoid medication

 c) Non steroidal Ibuprofen

d) Chlorpromazine

Answer: d

Explanation: Non steroidal anti inflammatory medication don't cause sedation. Phenothiazine can potentiate the sedative effect .

Question 35: **Anticipatory Grief, according to the nurse understanding is?**

 a) Short term

 b) Resolved

 c) Unacknowledged

 d) Unconscious process

Answer: d

Explanation: An unconscious process refers to sadness that is associated with a shock or sudden unhappy news. Generally anticipatory grief is associated with an unconscious process.

Question 36: **Louis receives total body irradiation for hematopoietic stem cell transplant. After one year he reports dullness in vision and ocular sensitivity. What is said to be the cause of above symptoms?**

 a) Optic neuritis

 b) Crossed eye

 c) Loss of vision

 d) Cataract

Answer: d

Explanation: Radiation can damage tissues by changing cell structure and damaging DNA. This can also lead to dimness in photophobia leading to Cataract.

Question 37: **William has been diagnosed with esophageal cancer. He suddenly reports having difficulty in swallowing and coughing. Which among the following will be considered more by the nurse?**

 a) Cavity

 b) Aspiration

 c) Dry mouth

 d) Acid reflex

Answer: b

Explanation: High risk of obstructive dysphagia in esophageal cancer generally leads to Aspiration.

Question 38: **Which of the following exemplifies complicated grief as demonstrated by the spouse of the patient who died recently?**

a) Seeking out new organization to join

b) Attending the support group for the family of cancer patients

c) Removing all the pictures from the house and refusing to discuss about the descendant

d) Avoiding discussion with hospice service

Answer: c

Explanation: Complicated grief is generally unresolved or it can take a long duration to resolve. This is caused due to the loss of a closest people or with whom they are living with. Therefore it better to stay away from having conversation about the descendant.

Question 39: **Catherine, suffering from ovarian cancer develops severe nausea ending up vomiting in large volume of fluids. This causes abdominal pain and rigid palpation with diminishing bowel sounds due to little bowel movements. She is not feverish but feels difficulty in breathing. The most preferred diagnosis is:**

a) Perforation of gastro intestinal tract

b) Colon Obstruction

c) Small Intestine Obstruction

d) Fecal impactions

Answer: c

Explanation: These are consistent symptoms of small intestine obstruction. Bowel obstruction occurs due to sudden and frequent nausea and vomiting in large volumes. Dexamethasone can relieve few symptoms as it reduces inflammation and swelling and also provides relief to nausea.

Question 40: Michelle is an advanced cancer patient. She is been taken care by her daughter at home. Her daughter states, " No one in my family understand how tiring cooking, cleaning and caring giving can be ". What will be most appropriate solution?

a) Visiting friends

b) Approaching support groups for caregivers

c) Visiting a psychologist

d) Attending motivation camps

Answer: b

Explanation: These feelings are very common among the care givers. So the best approach is caregiver support group. These groups can be therapeutic as they voice out these feelings. There are many online support groups also if they can't find any local support groups.

Question 41: **Which among the following will be the major side effects received by the patient due to the intake of irinotecan?**
 a) Patchy hair loss
 b) Diarrhea
 c) Expelling stomach content out of mouth forcefully
 d) Constriction of pupil of eye

Answer: b

Explanation: Irinotecan under the name of camptosar is a medication used to treat colon cancer, and small cell lung cancer. For colon cancer it is used either alone or with fluorouracil. For small cell lung cancer it is used with cisplatin. It is given by slow injection into a vein. About 35% of the people receiving this experience severe Diarrhea and neutropenia.

Question 42: **What combines with a mouse to form a cosmetic monoclonal antibody?**
 a) Pig antibody
 b) cow antibody
 c) Plant antibody
 d) Human antibody

Answer: d

Explanation: The mouse and human antibodies combine at a ratio of 70% human and 30% foreign antibodies. These are termed as chimeric monoclonal antibody.

Question 43: **Michelle after entering a palliative care underwent a treatment for leukemia that included chemotherapy. The Absolute Neutrophil Count is 526/ mm³, whereas her white blood cells close g is 5300/ mm³. Michelle has higher risk for which among the following options?**
 a) Fracture

b) Infection

c) Wheezing

d) Hypotension

Answer: b

Explanation: If the Absolute Neutrophil Count (ANC) falls below 1000mm³, then there is a chance of increase in risk rapidly. The normal neutrophil count of an adult is 1800 to 7700 mm³. Neutropenia occurs if the ANC decreases. Neutropenia is the severe complication in chemotherapy and other diseases such as leukemia. If a patient has both neutropenia and fever then the patient is prone to an infection that becomes life threatening.

Question 44: John has been evaluated for chronic leukemia. He has a history for cardiac disease reports of tachycardia and dyspnea. Which of the following blood cell count is most likely to indicate the cause?

a) Absolute neutrophils count - 1700/ mm³

b) White blood cells Count - 2960 mm³

c) Platelet count -1000,000 mm³

d) Level of Hemoglobin - 7.9 g/dl

Answer: d

Explanation: A condition in which the blood doesn't have enough healthy red blood cells is termed as anemia. Hgb level below 8g/dl is termed as severe anemia. Clinical signs are tachycardia, dyspnea at rest, angina, headache, and dizziness.

Question 45: Name the governmental organization which is responsible for the protection of human subjects and states that when performing studies involving human beings, the researcher must first obtain informed consent, in an easily understandable manner?

a) WHO

b) FDA

c) CDC

d) PAHO

Answer: b

Explanation: The FDA is responsible for the protection of human subjects and it demands that when performing studies involving people, the researcher must obtain informed consent in easily understandable language. The informed consent must include all the necessary details as stated by the FDA.

Question 46: Robin was provided with an adequate teaching in chemotherapy and Myelosuppression. He tries to demonstrate with his understanding. Which point is said to initiate his demonstration?

a) Myelosuppression refers to the immune system reaction of the body to a particular medicine.

b) Myelosuppression occurs when there is an elevation in the white blood cell count.

c) Myelosuppression is unintentional before blood transfusion

d) Myelosuppression is a potential side effects to many cancer treatments.

Answer: d

Explanation: The response of the immune system is decreased by causing neutropenia, anemia and thrombocytopenia during chemotherapy. This is generally referred as Myelosuppression. Therefore it is said to be the potential side effect of many cancer types.

Question 47: A patient is scheduled to receive oxaliplatin. Which of the following denotes that the patient needs additional teaching?

a) Before starting my chemotherapy I'm scheduled to get my first flu shot.

b) I'm going to eat ice chips while receiving chemotherapy in order to avoid mouth sores.

c) I'll call the triage number if I develop fever

d) I have ordered a wig to match my hair color

Answer: b

Explanation: When a patient is scheduled to receive Oxaliplatin, intake of ice chips and cold foods has to be avoided along with the fluids.

Question 48: Certain medications tend to interfere with cell membrane bound targets by blocking ligand receptor activation and immune modulation. Which of the following is considered as the interfering medication?

a) Anti-tumor antibiotics

b) Monoclonal antibody

c) Antineoplastic agent

d) Vascular permeability factor

Answer: b

Explanation: The rapid growth of the cancer cell can be prevented by the binding of monoclonal activity of the tumor cell and preventing the binding of ligand receptor by blocking other molecules from getting attached to the cells. Monoclonal antibody can therefore prevent the growth of the cancer cells.

Question 49: **The most likely cause of palmar plantar erythrodysesthesia is?**
a) Decreased circulation after infusion
b) Rupture of capillaries due to pressure and friction
c) Arranging for an occupational therapy
d) Over exposure of fast growing skin cells

Answer: b

Explanation: Palmar plantar erythro dysesthesia is due to rupture of capillaries that generally occur while walking, or due to any activities that involves bearing extra weight.

Question 50: **A patient has a visible skin sloughing and tissue breakdown. This is said to occur after Leakage of fluid (Extravasation). Which among the following is appropriate for the above causes?**
a) Application of ice pack
b) Consultation with plastic surgeon
c) Administering amoxicillin
d) Consultation with infectious disease

Answer: b

Explanation: After extravasation if a patient tends to have visible skin sloughing and breakdown of tissue then the patient must have a consultation with the plastic surgeon.

Question 51: **The condition that requires treatment by allogeneic stem cell transplant is?**
a) Hodgkin Lymphoma
b) Follicular thyroid cancer
c) Chronic Myeloid leukemia
d) Multiple myeloma

Answer: c

Explanation: By using allogeneic transplant, chronic myeloid leukemia can be treated.

Question 52: **The Carcinogenic medication among the following is?**
a) Streptozotocin
b) Etoposide
c) Furan

d) Anthraquinone

Answer: b

Explanation: Etoposide is well known as the human carcinogen. It is used in the treatment of testicular cancer lung cancer and lymphoma.

Question 53: **A patient has been diagnosed with lymphomatous meningitis. Which among the following will be the chemotherapy medication?**

a) Vincristine

b) Cytarabine

c) Acyclovir

d) Rifampicin

Answer: b

Explanation: Cytarabine, also known as cytosine arabinoside (ara-C), is a chemotherapy medication used to treat acute myeloid leukemia (AML), acute lymphocytic leukemia (ALL), chronic , leukemia (CML), and non-Hodgkin's lymphoma.

Question 54: **Until which situation should a hospice patient nearing death be offered food and water?**

a) As long as the patient wishes to consume food and water.

b) As long as the patient is conscious.

c) Until the patient begins hydration and artificial feeding.

d) Until the patient becomes lethargic.

Answer: a

Explanation: The patient should be given food and water until the patient begins to lose interest in it. The other options is not recommended because they bring unwanted pain and suffering to the dying patient.

Question 55: **A patient is receiving pain medication throughout the day as the patient was diagnosed with cognitive impairment and metastatic colon cancer. The nurse notes certain actions of patient: This includes short period of hyperventilation, frequent crying, fist clenched and lying rigidly and is increasingly combative. Which among the following matches the nurse suspicion?**

a) Increasing mental illness

b) Increasing antibiotics

c) Drowsiness due to pain killers

d) Pain control is not sufficient

Answer: d

Explanation: According to the Pain Assessment In Advanced Dementia (PAINAD) the patient is exhibiting non verbal indications of pain. These include negative in speech or speaking quietly, rapid breathing with increases pain, may be tensed, clenched fist , lying in fetal position and increasing combativeness.

Question 56: Among the following, which option can clearly explain the cancer survivorship plan?

a) Outlining about the expected follow up care after the treatment

b) Explaining about the medications

c) Exploring with the hospice care

d) Outlining about the primary therapies received during initial treatments

Answer: a

Explanation: By providing the patient with long term follow up care after treatment is the main aim of cancer survivorship plan. Appropriate schedule for screening, early and late effects of the treatments, description of the therapies are some of the other information included in the cancer survivorship plan.

Question 57: A patient is afebrile with generalized oral erythema, white patches on the palate, xerostomia and lump like sensation while swallowing after one week of chemotherapy. Which among the following can cure the above symptoms?

a) Amoxicillin

b) Pan endoscopy

c) Fluconazole

d) Paracetamol

Answer: c

Explanation: Fluconazole is an antifungal medicine that is used to cure oral candida with redness and with cottage cheese appearance.

Question 58: Temozolomide are used for administering certain brain cancer. What will be nurse advice to patient who is about to begin temozolomide medication?

a) Diarrhea is the common side effects

b) Neutropenia occurs after 22 to 28 days of completion

c) Uncommon side effects are nausea and vomiting

d) Weekly monitoring the amount of protein in urine is necessary

Answer: b

Explanation: As leukopenia and thrombocytopenia are dose limiting toxicities that are not cumulative, therefore treatment cycle is between 22 to 28 days and recovers within 14 days.

Question 59: Harry, with small cell lung cancer has observed the following changes; increase of weight up to 4 pounds, headache and excessive thirst. These are generally the symptoms of?

a) Hemolytic Uremic Syndrome (HUS)

b) Pericardial Tamponade

c) Tumor lysis syndrome

d) SIADH syndrome

Answer: d

Explanation: 80% reason for symptom of inappropriate anti-diuretic hormone syndrome (SIADH) is due to small cell lung cancer. Symptoms also include lethargy, muscle cramps and weakness.

Question 60: Proto-oncogenes can be described as?

a) The gene that makes tumor cells back to normal Genes

b) The gene that can provoke abnormal tumor growth

c) A gene that has the ability to become a transformer gene by transforming a normal cell into cancer cell

d) A gene that looks like a normal cell

Answer: c

Explanation: The gene that has a potential to cause abnormal cell growth are termed as oncogenes. When exposed to certain carcinogens, a gene that can become an oncogene is known as proto-oncogenes. They control the code that make proteins that help in differentiation and cell growth.

Question 61: Which of the following cancer type should be screened by 25 year old Michelle with BRCA1 mutation, who also underwent Bilateral Preventative

Mastectomies for Breast Cancer?

a) Lymphatic Cancer

b) Brain Cancer

c) Ovarian Cancer

d) Breast Cancer

Answer: c

Explanation: Using transvaginal ultrasound, BRCA1 or BRCA2 mutation patient must be screened every 6 months for ovarian cancer at the age of 25 along with Serum CA125 Level Checking. Michelle is advised for removal of ovaries and fallopian tube once she completes her child bearing or after 35 years of age.

Question 62: A patient is at her dying stage. Her daughter states that she wishes to do something for her mother's care , but she doesn't know what to do. How can the nurse help the patient's daughter?

a) By showing the daughter about the simple procedures such as mouth care

b) By saying that her presence is enough to make her mother happy

c) By telling her to have a peaceful conversation with her mother

d) By telling her not to disturb her mother

Answer: a

Explanation: Simple procedures such as teaching mouth care can make the daughter help her mother with her health care. This can respond to the daughter's request. During this period, the family members feel helpless as they can't see their loved ones dying. Therefore by giving tasks, can make them to feel needed. Having a peaceful conversation with her mother can also help but not according to her daughter's request.

Question 63: Mathew was diagnosed with intractable dyspnea. Even during the end of his life, he didn't find any relief with the traditional intervention. What will be the upcoming step considered by the nurse?

a) Informs the patient about the completion of all the therapies

b) Asks the physician to increase the dosage

c) Calls the anesthetist to increase the dosage of anesthesia

d) Discussing about the Palliative sedation initiated with the team.

Answer: d

Explanation: Palliative sedation is considered as end of the life therapy for Mathew when therapies such as IV opioids, oxygen, diuretics and benzodiazepines fails to give relief from the intractable dyspnea.

Question 64: A patient who has been enrolled in clinical trials has made an informed decision. Which among the following suitably match his informed decision?

a) The physician has explained all these to my family

b) Gained knowledge from cancer blog and came to know about its survival rate

c) Though there is no positive response from family, patient believes the process

d) Physician wouldn't have suggested if it was not suitable.

Answer: a

Explanation: The important duty and responsibility is to inform the consent. The decision made should not depend on others and the patient should have the freedom of choice.

Question 65: Robert's son insist that he will make all the decision regarding his father's care even though he is alert in making decisions. What will be the appropriate reply of the nurse?

a) To ask his son not to interfere in Robert's decision

b) To arrange a meeting with family members and health care members to discuss patient's wish

c) By allowing his son to make decisions

d) By suggesting motivation groups

Answer: b

Explanation: Robert has legal rights to decide so it is not advisable to address this issue directly to his son or family members as it may cause conflicts. So it is better to arrange meeting with the health care members and family members so that this issue can be explained clearly and also about the patient's wish.

Question 66: Which of the following disease can be cured by allogeneic stem cell transplant?

a) Breast Cancer

b) Lymphoma

c) Acute lymphoblastic leukemia

d) Germ cell tumors

Answer: c

Explanation: An allogeneic stem cell transplant uses healthy blood stem cells from a donor to replace the disease or damaged region. This can vary between myeloablative and non myeloablative. This can cure acute lymphoblastic leukemia.

Question 67: Which among the following can occur due to the negligence of attending a patient during their end of life?
a) Hopes to recovery
b) Premature death
c) Sense of peace
d) Adequate pain control
Answer: b
Explanation: Premature death includes suicide or losing all hopes of getting cured. Therefore it is important for the nurse to address the patient even during the end of their life.

Question 68: Robert, a patient with colon cancer underwent a bowel resection with colostomy. He suddenly experiences an abnormal finding on his third postoperative day. Which among the following matches his findings?
a) Moist bright, pink stoma
b) A dull, grey stoma
c) Air in the ostomy appliances
d) Slight stoma bleeding
Answer: b
Explanation: A moist reddish pink is said to be the normal condition of healthy stoma. Robert experiences a dull grey stoma due to lack of blood flow, ischemia or necrosis. In this case Robert has to immediately report to a physician.

Question 69: Which of the following medication is given for radiation induced diarrhea?
a) Glutamine
b) Loperamide
c) Erythromycin
d) Cetirizine
Answer: b
Explanation: Loperamide is a medication used to decrease the frequency of diarrhea. It is often used for this purpose in, inflammatory bowel disease, and short bowel syndrome. It is not recommended for those with blood in the stool, mucus in the stool or fevers.

Question 70: Cancer patients are generally given opioids to cure severe pains. When a patient suddenly complains about itching (pruritus), what can be done to manage this ?

a) Aspirin

b) Antipyretics

c) Celexa

d) Antihistamines

Answer: d

Explanation: Pruritus is generally caused due to release of histamine that can be managed by administrating anti histamines.

Question 71: Who is at the greater risk among the following for bone marrow depression after radiation treatment?

a) A 58-year-old patient who is receiving radiation for solitary liver metastasis

b) A 46-year-old patient receiving boost for Lumpectomy site

c) A 25-year-old patient receiving chemotherapy and radiation for Hodgkin lymphoma

d) A 67-year-old patient who is being treated for basal cell carcinoma of face

Answer: c

Explanation: Myelosuppression or bone marrow depression generally occurs for the patient who receives chemotherapy and also radiation treatment.

Question 72: Among the following, which one causes more blisters or is a vesicant?

a) Melphalan

b) Dactinomycin

c) Dalcabazine

d) Topotecan

Answer: b

Explanation: Metastatic testicular tumors (nonseminomatous), Gestational trophoblastic neoplasm, locally recurrent or loco regional solid tumors (sarcomas, carcinomas and adenocarcinomas) Soft tissue sarcoma are some of the cancer for which Dactinomycin will be administered. It is considered a vesicant.

Question 73: A patient is receiving Fluorouracil and leucovorin for an unresectable T2 N2 M1 adenocarcinoma of the colon. Which among the following is considered as the

goal for this treatment?

a) Increase in cellular contact inhibition

b) Promotion of cellular transformation

c) Radio sensitivity promotion

d) Control in cancer growth

Answer: d

Explanation: T2 N2 M1 is said to be the advanced metastatic cancer. It is said to be the stage 4 colon cancer. With an unresectable disease, cure is not possible. Until there is progression in disease, chemotherapy setting is given.

Question 74: Which among the following is described as the coping skill that rely on intrapsychic process?

a) Focusses only on problems

b) Focusing on appraisal

c) Focusses on emotion

d) Focusses only on avoidance

Answer: c

Explanation: In order to elicit emotions, feelings and concern, a person should rely upon the emotion focused skill that are associated with intrapsychic process.

Question 75: Michelle, who received cyclophosphamide five years ago for her breast cancer reported about the beginning of bruising and fatigue recently. These symptoms appears to be the suspect for which of the following options?

a) Liver failure

b) Secondary leukemia

c) Cardiomyopathy

d) Leukoencephalopathy

Answer: b

Explanation: While using alkylating agent the risk for having secondary leukemia increases for Michelle. Here the alkylating agent is cyclophosphamide.

Question 76: In order to screen the malignancy, which among the following tumor marker is used?

a) Prostate-specific antigens

b) CA-125

c) Carcinoembryonic antigen

d) Human chorionic gonadotropin

Answer: a

Explanation: Only prostate specific antigen marker can be used to test the malignant of cancer by screening.

Question 77: **What is the risk factor of development Lymphedema after the surgery for breast cancer?**

a) Leukoreduced

b) Low body mass index

c) Axillary node dissection

d) Somatic

Answer: c

Explanation: An axillary lymph node dissection (ALND) is surgery to remove lymph nodes from the armpit (underarm or axilla). The lymph nodes in the armpit are called axillary lymph nodes. Other symptoms include radiation, Obesity, lymphovascular invasion. This causes the risk of Lymphedema after breast cancer surgery.

Question 78: **What type of cancer can be prevented when oral contraceptive pills are consumed for more than 5 years?**

a) Endometrial cancer

b) Lung cancer

c) Breast cancer

d) Ovarian cancer

Answer: d

Explanation: Here oral contraceptive are recommended to aid in preventing the families from ovarian cancer, who have Lynch syndrome. Genetically they have no risk for breast cancer.

Question 79: **The type of cancer that can develop due to excessive use of smokeless tobacco and alcohol is?**

a) Lymphatic cancer

b) Lung cancer

c) Gastric cancer

d) Laryngeal cancer

Answer: d

Explanation: By using alcohol and smokeless tobacco together can cause Laryngeal cancer. It increases the risk of development up to to 50%.

Question 80: When a nurse has the ability to recognize and respect difference in beliefs, values and lifestyle, which among the following will the nurse try to demonstrate?
a) Presentation
b) Non maleficence
c) Protective buffering
d) Cultural competence

Answer: d

Explanation: Cultural competence generally refers to the identification of differences in the culture, beliefs and respect those differences among different people throughout their treatment duration.

Question 81: Before starting the process of chemotherapy, patient has to generally sign a consent form. He has a question regarding the treatment. What will the nurse do now?
a) Ensures of getting the consent form signed and beginning the treatment
b) Begins to administer while explaining the treatment
c) Asks the healthcare general to explain the treatment
d) Addresses patient's concerns before starting the treatment

Answer: d

Explanation: Initially nurse has to make the patient feel comfortable in asking question relating to treatment without any hesitation so that the patient can be relaxed without any unanswered questions.

Question 82: The most effective treatment for the severe pain that is associated with the post herpetic neuropathy is?
a) Dihydromorphinone
b) Extra strength acetaminophen
c) Amitriptyline
d) Propoxyphene

Answer: c

Explanation: Pain associated with herpes zoster is described as continuous, deep and burning which can be severe and deliberating. Treatment for acute herpes zoster is by using opioids. Treatment for post herpetic neuralgia is tricyclic antidepressants.

Question 83: The primary source of information by the patient while assessing the level of pain will be?
 a) Medication for current pain
 b) Self reporting
 c) Monitored Vital signs
 d) Medical diagnosis
Answer: b
Explanation: Assessment of pain intensity by the patient report is considered as the important consideration in determining medical treatment by the guidelines for cancer pain treatment from the Agency for Health Care Policy and Research, the American Pain Society, the National Comprehensive Cancer Network, and the World Health Organization (WHO).

Question 84: Richard has been diagnosed with advanced level of lung cancer. He reports having a rectum disorder, small amount of liquid stools and lower abdominal pain. The nurse will?
 a) Withhold all scheduled opioid until bowel function is restored.
 b) Provide a non-stimulating laxative
 c) Administer oral laxative and probiotic therapy
 d) Initiate a bulk forming laxative and force fluids
Answer: b
Explanation: In order to relieve severe or complete constipation, a non-stimulant laxative, glycerin suppository, or oil retention injection into the rectum can be administered.

Question 85: A patient suddenly reports the emergency department of having slurred speech, shuffling gait and Tremors while receiving prochloroperazine. Which of the following causes the above symptoms?
 a) Hypocalcemia
 b) Heart Attack
 c) Extrapyramidal reaction
 d) Psychomotor seizure

Answer: c

Explanation: Extrapyramidal symptoms, also called drug-induced movement disorders, describe the side effects caused by certain antipsychotic and other drugs. Extrapyramidal side effects include difficulty speaking or swallowing, loss of balance, shuffling gait or rigidity, twitching, or weakness of the arms and legs.

Question 86: A patient diagnosed with breast cancer was given a dose of IV doxorubicin an anthracycline DNA-binding agent. Soon the patient was observed to be suffering from symptoms like swelling, redness, itching and vesicles at IV insertion site. The course of action that the nurse should follow after discontinuing the medication is:
a) The nurse should apply some ice and administer dimethyl sulfoxide.
b) The nurse should apply some heat and administer dimethyl sulfoxide.
c) The nurse should apply some ice and administer dexrazoxane.
d) The nurse should apply some heat and administer dexrazoxane.

Answers : c

Explanation: The medications must be stopped as soon as the symptoms occur because vesicants such as anthracyclines cause local tissue damage and necrosis. The nurse must apply some ice to the area of administration to minimize the spread of the agent to the surrounding areas. The cold pack should be applied for 20 minutes for a minimum of four times daily for three days.

Question 87: After a loop electrosurgical excision procedures, what information will the nurse provide to the patient?
a) To avoid inserting anything into the vagina for 4 weeks
b) To expect extreme fatigue for several months
c) To Sit upright most of the time
d) To begin an exercise program to reduce weight gain

Answer: a

Explanation: It is advised to avoid inserting anything into the vagina for 4 weeks. It is normal to have some mild cramping, spotting, and dark or black-colored discharge for several days. The dark discharge is from the medicine applied to your cervix to control bleeding.

Question 88: In order to decrease the sleep disturbances, which of the following can be suggested?

a) Setting a comfortable bedroom temperature

b) Watching movies prior to bedtime.

c) Requesting the healthcare provider to stop treatment

d) Stretching in bed and doing moderate exercise

Answer: a

Explanation: Irrespective of the other factors, a comfortable room temperature before bedtime can stimulate a good sleep without any disturbance.

Question 89: What is the most common cause of lung cancer?

a) Exposure to direct or secondary tobacco smoke.

b) Genetic mutation.

c) Exposure to ultraviolet rays from the sun.

d) Exposure to chemical waste.

Answer: a

Explanation: Smoking is responsible for almost 90% of the total cases of lung cancer. Smoking is also responsible for various other types of cancer. All cancer patients are advised to discontinue the use of tobacco and they are also asked to quit smoking.

Question 90: Who has a higher risk of skin breakdown?

a) A patient with hyperpigmentation

b) A patient with decreased sensory perception

c) A patient with decreased serum albumin level

d) Higher mobilized patient

Answer: b

Explanation: Skin breakdown occurs when blood flow to your skin is limited or cut off altogether. Left untreated, skin breakdown can lead to infection, amputation or even death.

Question 91: Which among the following is said to be the suitable integrative modality for the patient who has pain with a platelet count of 12000/mm³?

a) Chemotherapy

b) Massage

c) Reiki therapy

d) Acupuncture

Answer: c

Explanation: Reiki is a form of alternative medicine called energy healing. Reiki practitioners use a technique called palm healing or hands-on healing through which a "universal energy" is said to be transferred through the palms of the practitioner to the patient in order to encourage emotional or physical healing. It would be appropriate for the patient with low platelet count.

Question 92: **What is best approach while helping a dying patient in completing a life review?**
a) By asking question without any hesitation in order to acquire more knowledge
b) By asking regular question
c) By having a comfortable conversation with the patient
d) By making a formal conversation with the family members

Answer: a

Explanation: The best approach is to make the patient talk freely. This is primarily an exercise for a dying patient to understand the meaning of life and relieve their lives. The nurse should generally question about the patient's childhood and gradually shifting the conversation with the patient's family members. The nurse can guide the patient by making this conversation a more interactive and ending by asking, " Have you done anything differently and exciting in your life? ".

Question 93: **Breast cancer survivor suddenly weeps to a nurse saying that she didn't expect that lymphedema would happen to her. How will the nurse react the patient?**
a) By allowing the patient to express her feelings
b) By assuring the quick recovery of lymphedema
c) By teaching the prevention methods of lymphedema recurrence
d) By taking a recent history to identify the occurrence of lymphedema

Answer: a

Explanation: Change in the body structure can affect the psychologically. So it is better to let the patient express her feelings so that nurse can acknowledge the patient's loss and encourage her expression.

Question 94: **Which of the following principles does advanced directives are based upon?**
a) Kindness

b) Autonomy

c) Justice

d) Truthfulness

Answer: b

Explanation: Advanced directives are generally based on the principle of autonomy. Every individual has an obligation to respect the autonomy of other persons, which is to respect the decisions made by other people concerning their own lives. This is also called the principle of human dignity.

Question 95: A patient with glioblastomas has been receiving radiation therapy. Which among the following would be the statement mentioned by the patient after understanding the teachings?

a) ' I shall avoid hair wash '

b) ' I can now stop taking steroids '

c)' I might experience permanent hair loss '

d) ' I shouldn't worry having a head ache. '

Answer: c

Explanation: Radiation therapy for glioblastomas can cause permanent hair loss. Other side effects include severe tiredness, trouble with memory and speech, skin and scalp changes.

Question 96: Which among the following statement correctly explains about the use of spouse as a translator for non-English speaking patient?

a) Translation by spouse can generally increase the patient's confidence level

b) Translation by the patients spouse is not recommended

c) Translation is allowed only when the spouse clear a qualification test

d) Translation is allowed only when the professional is not available

Answer: b

Explanation: Professional translators are suggested in order to avoid any conflicts due to inability of pronouncing the medical terms. Therefore patient's spouse are not recommended for translation.

Question 97: What will be the first step in oncology clinical setting using evidence based

practices?

a) Assess the patient need to define the problem

b) Using a medical model to explain the problems

c) Adding all the changes in care to experience the outcome

d) Before literature research, define the patient's outcome.

Answer: a

Explanation: Initial assessing of patient's needs, identifying appropriate resources and selecting process can change the evidences into practices.

Question 98: Which of the following is the primary measure to prevent cancer?

a) Guaiac fecal occult blood test

b) Usage of sunscreen

c) Systemic estrogens therapy

d) Self-examination of testicle

Answer: b

Explanation: Primary measure to prevent cancer is by using sunscreen. Other measures include immunization and Avoiding Consumption of tobaccos.

Question 99: The following are the symptoms of a patient suffering from stage IV Lung Cancer; Difficulty in differentiating between anginal pain (progressive dyspnea), facial swelling; swelling of neck, arms,hands and thorax due to the fluid from the tissue; Distended jugular,temporal and arm veins; disturbance in vision; headache and disorientation (altered mental status). The diagnosis for the above symptoms are:

a) Superior Vena Cava Syndrome (SVCS)

b) Lung embolism

c) Compression of Spinal Cord

d) Syndrome for Inappropriate secretion of Anti-Diuretic Hormone(SIADH)

Answer: a

Explanation: These are said to be the consistent symptoms of SVCS due to invasion or compression of SVC, that are also associated with other cancer types such as breast, brain, resulting in cerebral anoxia, obstruction in bronchi and Laryngeal Edemas (at extreme cases) which can be treated by radiation, chemotherapy and surgery. Oxygen Therapy and corticosteroids are considered as supportive measures at extreme cases.

Question 100: For muscle invasive bladder cancer which among the following is said to be the primary goal?

a) Preventing the development to brain

b) Preparing the body for chemotherapy

c) Reducing the surgery time

d) Preserving the bladder function

Answer: d

Explanation: Bladder function can be preserved in the case of muscle invasive bladder cancer during radiotherapy. This does not compromise the long term disease specific survival.

Question 101: Which of the following conditions are included in Myeloablation for transplanting stem cell?

a) Growth analysis

b) Nutritional analysis

c) High dose chemotherapy

d) Retrograde surgical intervention

Answer: c

Explanation: Myeloablation refers to total body irradiation that prevents autologous hematologic recovery. By administering high dosage of chemotherapy, residual disease can be eliminated prior to hematopoietic stem cell transplant.

Question 102: Cherry is a survivor of Malignant Melanoma. She has completed her treatment one year ago, but still complains about tiredness. Which among the following stimulants does the nurse foretell?

a) Lorazepam

b) Darbepoetin Alfa

c) Pegfilgrastim

d) Methylphenidate

Answer: d

Explanation: Methylphenidate is said to be one of the prominent psychostimulants used with the patients with malignant melanoma and also with advanced level of Cancer. This is said to report any improvement in cancer related symptoms but still under research level.

Question 103: What has to be done when Robin reports of yellow, crusted papules and

itching of shoulder after a targeted therapy?

a) Dilute hot bath water with half strength Dakin's solution

b) Apply lotion with Dimethicone

c) Using a moisturizer containing retinoid twice a day

d) Apply aloe Vera on the affected region

Answer: b

Explanation: Dimethicone is used as a moisturizer to treat or prevent dry, rough, scaly, itchy skin and minor skin irritations such as skin burns from radiation therapy. These are substances that soften and moisturize the skin and decrease itching and flaking.

Question 104: **Jonas, 62 years old patient with CD33 positive acute myeloid leukemia has a left ejection fraction of 40% during first relapse. What is the treatment suggested for Jonas?**

a) All trans retinoic acids

b) Gemtuzumab ozogamicin

c) Cytosine arbinoside

d) Intravenous drug Rituximab

Answer: b

Explanation: Patients who are not considered for cytotoxic chemotherapy are administered with Gemtuzumab ozogamicin usually above 60 years of age.

Question 105: **In what ways does the cancer cell differ from the ordinary cells?**

a) Cancer cells divide only when the older cells are destroyed

b) Cancer cells migrate to the neighboring locations and tissues

c) Ordinary cells generally reside in new areas

d) Ordinary cells doesn't allow contact with the other cells

Answer: b

Explanation: Cancer cells are cells that divide relentlessly, forming solid tumors or flooding the blood with abnormal cells. Cell division is a normal process used by the body for growth and repair. They are characterized by uncontrolled movement and abnormal growth.

Question 106: **Robert, a 19 year old patient diagnosed with testicular cancer fears about his potency to conceive children as he will be receiving cisplatin and pelvic radiation. What will be suggested for Robert by the nurse?**

a) Cryopreservation after completion of cisplatin treatment

b) Preserving the sperm before initiating the treatment

c) Sexual counseling throughout the treatment

d) After the completion of the treatment, sildenafil is given to patient before engaging into sexual activity.

Answer: b

Explanation: Sperm banking is recommended before initiating the treatment with cisplatin and pelvic radiation. This is because chemotherapy with cisplatin and alkylating agents can cause permanent infertility (Azoospermia). For future paternity Robert is suggested with sperm banking.

Question 107: NIOSH approved respirator should be worn for which of the following activity?

a) Penetrating an intravenous bag

b) While handling bodily fluids

c) Cleaning hazardous drug spill

d) While Administering an IV chemotherapeutic agent

Answer: c

Explanation: NIOSH approval is issued only to a specific and complete respirator assembly after the respirator has been evaluated in the laboratory and found to comply with all of the requirements of Title 42, Code of Federal Regulations , Part 84, and after the manufacturer's quality plan is determined to be satisfactory. This type of approved respirators are used while cleaning up hazardous drug spill.

Question 108: What will be the common adverse effect of a patient diagnosed with prostate cancer when treated with diethylstilbestrol?

a) Pneumonia

b) Gynecomastia

c) Arthritis

d) Bowel obstruction

Answer: b

Explanation: An enlargement or swelling of breast tissues in male is known as gynecomastia. This is a common effect of androgen deprivation therapy. This is due to the impaired balance of the estrogen and testosterone. Orchiectomy and Administering luteinizing hormone releasing hormone (LHRH) are other androgen deprivation method.

Question 109: A patient who is at the dying state experiences delirium. Medication that can manage this symptom will be?
a) Cetirizine
b) Haloperidol
c) Aprepitant
d) Paracetamol
Answer: b
Explanation: Haloperidol is used to manage delirium. It is also used in the treatment of schizophrenia, tics in Tourette syndrome, mania in bipolar disorder, nausea and vomiting, delirium, agitation, acute psychosis.

Question 110: William suddenly got provoked with a doubt while Docetaxel was infused. He asked the nurse why dexamethasone is prescribed. The nurse responds by saying that it prevents ?
a) Fatigue
b) Sudden uncontrolled electric disturbances
c) Fluid retention
d) Anorexia nervosa
Answer: c
Explanation: Dexamethasone is used as it prevents fluid retention. It is also used to reduce inflammation and suppress (lower) the body's immune response. It is used with other drugs to treat the following types of cancer: Leukemia. Lymphoma.

Question 111: What is the major benefit of survivorship care plan?
a) It allows the patient to make discussion with their oncologist after the completion of treatment.
b) It will be easier to monitor patient regarding side effects
c) It allows the patient to have medication during chemotherapy
d) It provides a clear idea about the care and surveillance after treatment
Answer: d
Explanation: Survivorship care plan has the following benefits to the patient: It shall provide complete information regarding the treatment received, the long term effects and the healthy choice of lifestyle and screenings throughout their life term.

Question 112: A patient with cancer experiences an erectile dysfunction. Which type of intervention is more likely to assist the patient?

a) Psychotherapy

b) Kegel exercise

c) Herbal dietary fibers

d) Oral phosphodiesterase type 5 inhibitors

Answer: d

Explanation: Certain studies state that patients can get cured with erectile dysfunction when they are assisted with oral phosphodiesterase type 5 inhibitors.

Question 113: How can the points be focused on the adults who have low literacy rate, during the cancer education programs?

a) Explaining the process with cartoon type illustration.

b) By providing information in the form of quiz

c) Explaining with medical term for better understanding

d) Repeating the same message in different form.

Answer: d

Explanation: For the adults who have low literacy levels find it easier to understand and also gets registered with the information easily when they are familiarized with the same message through different methodologies that include pictures, demonstrations, etc.

Question 114: William experiences extensive metastasis. He says, " I don't want any treatment. Anyways I'm going to die let me spend my time with my family". What will be the intervention of the nurse?

a) " You will definitely feel better tomorrow"

b) " Would you like to discuss about the hospice service?"

c)" Completing your treatment is more important"

d) " Did you discuss this with your support group?'

Answer: b

Explanation: Every patient who gets diagnosed with cancer becomes more emotional. They end up getting depressed when they feel that their treatment is getting exhausted or when they have lost the energy mentally to fight against the deadly illness. Here, William might feel hesitant about asking the hospice care. The nurse explains William that hospice care is not only just a care philosophy but it is place they are generally taken to.

Question 115: Which of the following should the patient follow while receiving intraperitoneal cisplatin?
a) Nothing has to be taken orally for 12 hours prior to treatment
b) Changing the position frequently while receiving medication
c) Medication has to be received under fluoroscopy
d) Medication has to be cold
Answer: b
Explanation: Repositioning from side to side for every 15 minutes during dwell time is being suggested by the nursing care management of the patient receiving intraperitoneal drug administration.

Question 116: What is the common side effect of palanosetron?
a) Hiccups
b) Itchiness
c) Constipation
d) Disturbance in mental ability
Answer: c
Explanation: Palanosetron is generally used in the prevention and treatment of chemotherapy-induced nausea and vomiting. The common side effects include Headache, constipation or diarrhea.

Question 117: Which among the following is the symptom exhibited by the newly diagnosed acute myeloid leukemia?
a) Palpitation
b) Headache
c) Petechiae
d) Pruritus
Answer: c
Explanation: The symptoms that are likely to occur with the patient who is newly diagnosed with acute myeloid leukemia is petechiae. Petechiae is generally termed by tiny round, brown-purple spots due to bleeding under the skin, may be in a small area due to minor trauma, or widespread due to blood-clotting disorder.

Question 118: William is taking opioids for pain management. He reported of increased

constipation and has started bowel retaining. What is said to be the best time to assist him to sit on a toilet or commode to initiate bowel evacuation?

a) Exactly before going to sleep

b) Early in the morning

c) About half an hour after meal

d) Whenever the patient urges to defecate

Answer: c

Explanation: It is better to assist William with scheduled defecation every day and about half an hour after every meal. This is because it helps to stimulate the gastro colic reflex that propels the fecal matter through colon. This can be sometimes stimulated by any stimulus but the usage has to be minimized during the progressive days. William has to maintain a proper record about his stool evacuation and its consistency.

Question 119: Michele is using fentanyl patches to control her pain caused due to ovarian cancer. She reports the nurse regarding the following symptoms; Difficulty in urinating and able to pass only small amount of urine. Bladder is not distended and has bilateral pain in the flank areas. Recent blood test reports shows slight hyperkalemia and is afebrile. These symptoms are due to?

a) Infection in bladder

b) Cervical cancer

c) Obstruction in upper urinary tract

d) Side effects caused by the intake of opioids

Answer: c

Explanation: The cause of urine retention is due to the obstruction in the upper urinary tract. This appears secondary to the ovarian cancer. Michele is likely to developed uremia if she is unable to drain her urine as her ureters are obstructed. This is associated with hyperkalemia. The bladder tends to fill normally and gets distended with pain with any bladder injection or opioids induced deficiency of detrusor muscle contraction.

Question 120: What will be the primary nursing intervention of the patient who develops grade 3 peripheral neuropathy?

a) Monitor serum electrolytes

b) Obtain an order for corticosteroids

c) To teach about safe home environment

d) Recommend for increased narcotic analgesia

Answer: c

Explanation: Symptoms for peripheral 3 neuropathy includes gradual onset of numbness, prickling or tingling in your feet or hands, which can spread upward into your legs and arms. Sharp, jabbing, throbbing or burning pain. Extreme sensitivity to touch. Therefore it is mandatory to teach proper home environments.

Question 121: In order to determine acute changes in nutritional status and also to monitor the dietary status of patient with cachexia, test are generally taken. Which of the following is most commonly monitored ?

a) Transferrin

b) Albumin and Globulin

c) Prealbumin

d) Albumin

Answer: c

Explanation: Prealbumin or transthyretin is monitored to determine changes in nutritional status. Prealbumin is said to be measured as it shows drastic decrease in level when there is a change in nutritional level. Albumin are said to be sensitive for long term protein deficiency rather than short term deficiency.

Question 122: A patient with prostate cancer experiences metastasis. Which among the following is said to metastasize frequently?

a) Brain

b) Liver

c) Bone

d) Lung

Answer: c

Explanation: Bone is said to be the frequent site for occurrence of metastasis whereas Liver and Lung experiences rare spread of metastatic effect.

Question 123: A Fluorouracil based chemotherapy combination has been administered to Ron, who has been employed as a landscaper. Which among the following symptom is most likely to occur?

a) Pulmonary toxicity

b) Gouty arthritis

c)Accumulation of fluid in lower limbs

d) Photosensitivity

Answer: d

Explanation: Anti-cancer medications and medications used to reduce side effects may contribute to the development of some eye problems such as photosensitivity.

Question 124: **A gay man is at the dying stage because of leukemia. He asked the hospice not to allow his parents to meet him in his room as his parents didn't accept his lifestyle or his partner. What will be best action done by the nurse?**

a) The nurse can ask his parents to leave a message as they are not allowed to meet him

b) The nurse can request the patient to meet his parents

c) The nurse informs his parents about his unwillingness to meet them

d) The nurse can talk with the hospice

Answer: a

Explanation: The best action done by the nurse is to request the parents to leave a message for his son as it is a right of the patient to deny them from meeting him. The nurse cannot directly say the reason to the parents as it causes more worries to his parents. The nurse cannot either request the patient as it is his choice or talk with the hospice regarding this.

Question 125: **Rosie, a 60-year-old obese diabetic patient is experiencing bleeding due to post menopause. Which of the following type of cancer is likely to occur in Rosie?**

a) Fallopian tube

b) Cervical

c) Ovary

d) Endometrial

Answer: d

Explanation: The other risk factors of endometrial cancer generally include hypertension, diabetes and development of menopause after the age of 52 years.

Question 126: **Restlessness, insomnia, diarrhea, heart palpitations, and irritability are the reactions expressed by newly diagnosed cancer patient. Patient also gets nervous and worried and asks for some medication for nerves. What will be the best response**

from the nurse?

a) Instructs the patient to ask for a sedative from the physician.

b) Informs the patient about the initiation of treatment

c) Ask the patient to explain his feelings further

d) Assure that the reason is due to cancer diagnosis

Answer: c

Explanation: Before treating anxiety, it is important to know the causes of anxiety. The nurse must help in identifying the cause of anxiety as it has several risk factors.

Question 127: Robin experiences persistent depressive disorder (dysthymic behavior) for several weeks. What should the nurse assess initially?

a) Depression

b) Bowel Habits

c) Recurrence of disease

d) Cognitive learning

Answer: a

Explanation: Cancer patients are generally said to stay stronger as they might experience depression which leads to poor outcome.

Question 128: Mild ascites along with increase in weight and early satiety were the complaints reported by the recently diagnosed lung cancer patient. There is a possibility of developing malignant ascites. Which among the following improves the risk?

a) Renal disease

b) Diabetes

c) Pulmonary Disease

d) Diverticulitis

Answer: a

Explanation: Patient with primary condition of liver, renal and cardiac disease are more bound to higher risk of ascites.

Question 129: What will be the initiation taken by the nurse when a patient complains about urticaria and pruritus while getting paclitaxel infused?

a) Administering diphenhydramine

b) Obtaining vital signs and monitor patients

c) Applying ice packs to the affected region.

d) The infusion of the medication has to be stopped

Answer: d

Explanation: Urticaria also known as hives are generally referred as skin rashes. The immediate step taken by the nurse when the patient complains about any hypersensitive allergy is to stop the infusion of medication.

Question 130: The patient has sudden dyspnea, wheezing, hypotension, throat and face swelling during the administration of chemotherapeutic agent intravenously. What will be the initial action of the nurse?

a) To stop administering oxygen
b) To decrease antihistamine
c) To discontinue the administering of chemotherapeutic agent
d) To increase administering epinephrine

Answer: c

Explanation: The nurse should immediately discontinue the chemotherapeutic agent and monitor the patients respiratory and cardiovascular status as these symptoms are persistent with anaphylaxis. Dyspnea is generally treated with higher oxygen concentration and once the patient gets stabilized the corticosteroids and antihistamines can be administered in order to prevent the recurrence and to treat Urticaria and swelling.

Question 131: Certain population is at the risk for the under treatment of pain during their end of the life. Which among the following correctly matches?

a) Younger adults
b) Elderly people
c) Diabetic patient
d) Men

Answer: b

Explanation: Any disease which has serious symptoms can be cured only when diagnosed at the earlier stage. Individual who are at higher risk for under treatment of any pain symptoms are generally women and elder people.

Question 132: Which of the following is considered as a modal quality of cancer treatment regarding surgery?

a) It causes less toxicity when used along with chemotherapy

b) It is considered as the only treatment that the patient requires

c) It is used as a palliative measure to relieve symptoms

d) It aims to remove only a portion of tumor

Answer: b

Explanation: Cancer surgery generally removes the tumor and the nearby tissue during an operation. It is one among the oldest treatment but it is still effective.

Question 133: The cells from which oligodendroglia tumors originate maintains the function of ?

a) Synovial fluid

b) Pericardial fluid

c) Myelin sheath

d) Cell body

Answer: c

Explanation: Oligodendroglia create myelin sheaths for CNS axons, paralleling the function of Schwann cells in the peripheral nervous system. It generally develops and maintains the Myelin sheath.

Question 134: A patient refuses to take opioids stating that even pain is a part of life. What will be the nurse response to this statement?

a) Exploring the meaning of pain with the patient

b) Schedule a visit with CanSurmount volunteer

c) Requesting an evaluation from the pain service

d) Referring pain to chaplain

Answer: a

Explanation: Pain is generally considered as punishment therefore the nurse helps in confronting the family about this opinion and brings positive mind.

Question 135: Richard is learning about patient controlled analgesia (PCA) pump from his nurse. Even though his nurse taught him the process at least for 3 times, he kept asking the same doubts repeatedly. The nurse also provides Richard with a pamphlet but he doesn't look at it at all. He says that he can't understand anything by looking at the pamphlet and doesn't know what to do next. What will be the next step taken by the nurse?

a) By allowing the patient to practice with the kit

b) By asking another nurse to teach him

c) By suggesting other alternative methods

d) By starting her teaching after some rest time

Answer: a

Explanation: A learning style which involves physical activities rather than listening or viewing pamphlet is known as tactile learning method or kinesthetic learning method. Since Richard is unable to understand oral teaching and through visual reading, it is better that he is allowed to learn manually. He can understand by operating the pump with minimal directions and maximum hands on experience.

Question 136: A patient has developed a wheel and pain at peripheral IV site during infusion of Doxorubicin. Which among the following is said to be an appropriate intervention?

a) Heat application

b) Administering mesnex

c) Applying hydrocortisone

d) Administering dexrazoxane

Answer: d

Explanation: By Administering dexrazoxane, pain and swelling at peripheral IV site during infusion of Doxorubicin can be controlled. This is generally due to extravasation.

Question 137: Charles has been diagnosed with invasive ductal adenocarcinoma of pancreas. Upon diagnosis, the disease most likely:

a) Metastatic to Cartilage

b) Remains without spreading to other body parts

c) Demonstrates the spread to liver

d) Displays the widespread fat globules

Answer: c

Explanation: Invasive ductal carcinoma (IDC), sometimes called infiltrating ductal carcinoma, is the most common type of breast cancer. About 80% of all breast cancers are invasive ductal carcinomas. Invasive means that the cancer has "invaded" or spread to the surrounding tissues. It also demonstrates the spread to liver.

Question 138: Which among the following reference will assist the nurse in determining the characteristics and safe handling precautions of medicine about which the nurse is concerned as being hazardous?

a) The Joint Commission Hospital Patient Safety Goals

b) NIOSH List of Antineoplastic and Other Hazardous Drug in Healthcare Setting

c) National Comprehensive Cancer Network Clinical Practice Guidelines in Oncology

d) The Joint Commission Hospital Patient Safety Goals

Answer: b

Explanation: NIOSH is known as National Institute for Occupational Safety and Health. It maintains the list of Antineoplastic and other hazardous drugs in the healthcare settings. It also consist of personal protective equipment required for safe handling and administration.

Question 139: For which of the practice standard of oncology nursing society should the nurse demonstrate behavioral consent for taking oncology certified nurse examination?

a) Ethical behavior

b) The extent to which the healthcare services are provided to the individual

c) Performance review

d) Professional performance

Answer: d

Explanation: In order to display professionalism, a voluntary action is performed by the nurse so that nurse will receive a professional certification.

Question 140: While treating with interleukin-2, which among the following is said to respond?

a) Advanced testicular cancer

b) Metastatic melanoma

c) Accumulation of abnormal B lymphocyte

d) Urothelial carcinoma

Answer: b

Explanation: When a patient is treated with interleukin 2 only Metastatic melanoma is said to respond. This is because it produce anti-cancer response rates of 15% to 20%.

Question 141: Which among the following is considered as the most important criteria for selecting the patient to participate in the phase 2 clinical trial?

a) The patient must have physiological diseases

b) The patient must have an adequate performance status

c) The patient should not be exposed to any chemotherapy treatment before.

d) The patient exhausted all approved treatments

Answer: b

Explanation: The characteristics that are considered for a phase 2 clinical trial are good performance status, minimal exposure to chemotherapy and the patient must have specific diagnosis. The response rate is considered as the primary endpoint of stage 2 clinical phase.

Question 142: William requires chronic platelet transfusions may develop antibodies and require further products to be:

a) Low body mass index

b) Reduced volume

c) Delayed

d) Leukoreduced

Answer: d

Explanation: Leukoreduction is the removal of white blood cells (or leukocytes) from the blood or blood components supplied for blood transfusion. After the removal of the leukocytes, the blood product is said to be Leukoreduced. Leukoreduced platelets are indicated for patients expecting multiple platelet transfusions to reduce the incidence of alloimmunization.

Question 143: Unilateral orchiectomy was scheduled for William who has testicular cancer. He enquires the nurse about his reproduction activities. What will be the response of nurse to William?

a) 50% reduction in fertility

b) Azoospermia

c) No change in fertility

d) Oligospermia

Answer: c

Explanation: William will not experience any changes as there will be no alteration due to removal of one testis and for a person who undergoes unilateral orchiectomy.

Question 144: William, a patient with prostate cancer administers oxycodone orally for

the relief from pain every 4 hours. A Nurse, while paying a home visit finds that there has been no bowel movement with constant and dull back pain for the past 3 days. These symptoms are likely to indicate?

a) Adverse effect of oxycodone

b) Excess abdominal fluid (Ascites)

c) Hypocalcemia

d) Impending spinal cord compression

Answer: d

Explanation: Tumor invades into the vertebrae causing collapse on the spinal cord that results in impending spinal cord compression. High risk for compression is generally for the patients with prostate cancer. Dull back pain is known to be the earlier symptom of spinal cord compression.

Question 145: Adjunct treatment option for neuropathy has been suggested by the thalidomide receiving patient. The suggestion given by the nurse based on the current evidence would be ?

a) Glutathione

b) Anticonvulsant medication Lamotrigine

c) Fish oil

d) Acupuncture

Answer: d

Explanation: The use of Acupuncture as the effective adjunct treatment for neuropathy has been reported by the evidences.

Question 146: What type of chemotherapy induced nausea does the patient experience after four days of chemotherapy?

a) Acute

b) Prolonged

c) Delayed

d) Refractory

Answer: c

Explanation: After chemotherapy, certain side effects are being experienced by the patients. One such side effect is delayed Nausea, which occurs within 24 hours of chemotherapy and lasts up to 5 days.

Question 147: Weight loss, abdominal pain and diarrhea are some of the symptoms

reported by Harry who is 70 years old. He also reported that these symptoms often interrupts his sleep. Harry's brother was recently diagnosed for prostate cancer. What will the nurse suspect?

a) Spastic colon

b) Klinefelter syndrome

c) Carcinoid syndrome

d) Neurofibromatosis

Answer: c

Explanation: Carcinoid syndrome occurs when a rare cancerous tumor called a carcinoid tumor secretes certain chemicals into your bloodstream, causing a variety of signs and symptoms. Generally patients with age above 65 who have close relative relatives diagnosed with prostate cancer are said to have a higher risk for the development of neuroendocrine tumor and carcinoid syndrome.

Question 148: After two weeks of chemotherapy, a patient reports bleeding gums and increased bruises even though the patient has normal platelet count. What is appropriate intervention to be done by the nurse?

a) Review the patient's medical report

b) Suggest the patient to have iron rich food

c) Reassure the patient that this symptoms will reduce after few days

d) Review the patient's history for prior treatment with ionizing radiation

Answer: a

Explanation: Some of the prescribed drugs can affect the platelet function and must be reviewed. This is because sometimes these symptoms with normal platelet count may suggest another cause.

Question 149: Paresthesia and dysesthesia (abnormal sensation) to hands, feet and mouth are caused by which of the following medication?

a) Ifex

b) Busulfan

c) Ifosfamide

d) Oxaliplatin

Answer: d

Explanation: Paresthesia and dysesthesia of hands, feet and mouth are caused by Oxaliplatin. Also known as Eloxatin, is a cancer medication used to treat colorectal cancer.

Question 150: Michelle, a patient has a negative result for BRCA mutation but her sister Rosie has a positive result. What kind of emotion does Michelle exhibit when she says with tears," I was always the troublesome kid"?
a) Survivor Guilt
b) Siblings rivalry
c) Transmitter guilt
d) Reactive Depression
Answer: a
Explanation: Michelle will be in a state where she is most likely to relate characters along with the test results. Survivor guilt occurs when a person tests negative and feel guilty as to why they were fortunate enough to test negative when a dear one tested positive.

Question 151: Radiation therapy is given to the patient with a tumor on the floor of the mouth. What advice is given to the patient?
a) Avoid using topical anesthetic
b) Avoid consuming alcohol
c) Avoid using less spices
d) Consume only less fluid everyday
Answer: b
Explanation: Consumption of alcohol can lead to burning sensation of the mouth. It may also delay the healing process.

Question 152: The nurse observes a raised pearly lesions on the patient's upper chest after completing the physical examination. Which among the following shows the above symptom?
a) Carcinoid syndrome
b) Pneumonitis
c) A basal cell carcinoma
d) Lung cancer
Answer: c
Explanation: Basal cells produce new skin cells as old ones die. Limiting sun exposure can help prevent these cells from becoming cancerous. Other symptoms include lesion, redness, loss of color, small bump, swollen blood vessels in the skin, or ulcers.

Question 153: Charles, a 21 year old cancer patient suddenly withdrew from college due to cancer resurrection. His family informs the nurse about his mood swings and refusal to meet his friends. What will be strategy achieved by the nurse initially?

a) Re enrolling in college courses
b) Clinical trial participation
c) Recognizing self-destructive behavior
d) Maintaining open communication

Answer: d

Explanation: Only when Charles starts to communicate with his family and friends, he shall be able to feel the support and value for his feeling through his communication so that he can be little better.

Question 154: Which among the following should the nurse focus while considering rehabilitation principle in a cancer patient?

a) Encouraging more rest periods
b) Focusing more on disabilities
c) Develop group goals
d) Emphasize capabilities

Answer: D

Explanation: Emphasizing functioning Vs dysfunction and capability Vs disabilities are certain rehabilitation principle. Balancing activity and rest time also emphasize the capability.

Question 155: Mathew, a 78 year old patient has been diagnosed with prostate cancer and cardiovascular disease. He has been administered with naproxen twice a day along with a daily dose of acetylsalicylic acid. What will be the instruction given to the patient?

a) Consulting the physician regarding the addition of cytoprotectants
b) About the increase in swelling during evening times
c) Consumption of medicine only in the empty stomach
d) To consume every medicine with proper time interval

Answer: a

Explanation: Naproxen is a nonsteroidal anti-inflammatory drug used to treat pain. Cytoprotection is a process by which the chemical compounds provide protection to the cells from the damage created by harmful agents. It is advisable to consult a physician regarding the cytoprotectants.

Question 156: **What is the most effective team size while developing multidisciplinary team?**
a) 12- 16 members
b) 1- 5 members
c) 12- 15members
d) 11- 20 members
Answer: b
Explanation: Important elements to be considered while developing a multidisciplinary teams are as follows: A team consists of less than 10 members. Every team member should have an individual skills that encloses problem solving, technical, interpersonal skills, decision making skills, etc., The team should be unified while performing a specific task. The teams members are accountable together rather than individually.

Question 157: **Persistent nausea, muscle cramps, weakness, and paresthesia of the fingers two days after receiving the first cycle of chemotherapy are the symptoms reported by the patient with Lymphatic cancer or lymphoma. Which among the following is experienced by the patient?**
a) Tumor lysis syndrome
b) Syndrome of anti-diuretic secretion hormone
c) Hypercalcemia
d) Disseminated intra vascular coagulation/ consumptive coagulopathy
Answer: a
Explanation: Metabolic imbalance that occurs with the rapid release of intracellular potassium, phosphorus, and nucleic acid into the blood as a result of killing of tissue is known as Tumor lysis syndrome. Muscle cramps, weakness, nausea and vomiting, diarrhea, lethargy, and paresthesia are the early signs and symptoms.

Question 158: **Before initiating the opioid therapy for Pain control, what order does the nurse anticipate initially?**
a) Treating occasional constipation
b) Stimulant laxative

c) Suppositories

d) Bulk laxative (Metamucil)

Answer: b

Explanation: Stimulant laxatives plus a stool softener is recommended when initiating opioid therapy as constipation is the most common side effect of opioid therapy.

Question 159: **According to the Buddhist tradition, they believe that a deceased person's body should not be disturbed for at least four hours. The most likely reason behind this might be:**

a) The person might have been diagnosed with an infectious disease and they might need some time to dispose the body properly.

b) They believe that a soul needs some time to leave off the body and be at peace.

c) The patient's family might need some time to cope-up with the patient's loss.

d) The patient's family may need some time to do the final rituals of the patient for his well-being in the afterlife.

Answer: b

Explanation: The Buddhists leave the body undisturbed for a long period of time because they believe that a soul needs some time to leave the body and be at peace. The Buddhists believe in multiple lifetimes like the Hindus and they also believe that the actions of their past lives might affect their present one. They call this as karma.

Question 160: **Among the following, which phase requires data monitoring committee for clinical trials?**

a) 5

b) 3

c) 2

d) 1

Answer: c

Explanation: A data monitoring committee (DMC), also called a data and safety monitoring board (DSMB) is an independent group of experts who monitor patient safety and treatment efficacy data while a clinical trial is ongoing. DMC is required for the third trial phase in order to protect the safety of trial patient.

Question 161: Mark who has colon mesothelioma has been scheduled for chemotherapy which is to be administered in the peritoneal space. Which is the type of device through which Mark attends his chemotherapy?

a) Intraventricular catheter reservoir (Ommaya reservoir)
b) Large diameter silicon port implantation
c) Insertion of central catheter peripherally
d) Arterial Catheter

Answer: B

Explanation: In order to deliver high amount of chemotherapy, intraperitoneal catheters or implanted ports are preferred highly for the patients with metastatic cancer into the abdomen and peritoneum, diagnosing ovarian cancer or colon mesothelioma or malignant ascites.

Question 162: The ethnic group that has high risk for developing cancer in Male is?

a) Pacific islanders
b) Asian Americans
c) African Americans
d) White Americans

Answer: c

Explanation: The ethics group that has the highest risk for cancer development in Male is African American males. The lower risk is generally for the Pacific islanders. Generally females have a lower risk of developing cancer than males among the ethnic groups. The African Americans and Caucasian (White Americans)have the highest death rates among both the males and females.

Question 163: List the two types of cancer for which hormone therapy is effective?

a) Liver and lymphoma
b) Breast and prostate
c) Leukemia and breast
d) Liver and prostate

Answer: b

Explanation: Success rates of hormonal therapy has been observed by treating breast cancer and prostate cancer.

Question 164: Among the following which is considered as the risk factor for the treatment related to pneumonitis?

a) Usage of steroids continuously

b) Lowering the concentration of oxygen therapy

c) For age less than 60 years

d) Mantle field radiation

Answer: d

Explanation: When having large volume of lung is included in the treatment field, the risk factor of pneumonitis is also increased.

Question 165: Why are certain tumor cells described as undifferentiated cells?

a) Because they grow at a faster rate

b) Because they resemble normal cells

c) Because they don't grow

d) Because they remain in same position

Answer: a

Explanation: Microscopic examination of the cell is required by the histologic headings in order to explain their resemblance as normal cells. These cells usually grow and spread at a normal rate. But the cells which are undifferentiated tend to be more aggressive and they spread more easily. They also grow rapidly. These cells are known as tumor cells . Every tumor cell has it's own level , higher the grade the more aggressive it becomes.

Question 166: What will be the response of the nurse when enquired about the risk of Lymphedema after undergoing breast conservation surgery with sentinel lymph node biopsy procedure and radiation?

a) If Lymphedema guidelines are followed then there will be no occurrence

b) If there is no development in the first year, then there is no development in the progressive years.

c)Although the risk is low precaution has to be taken

d) There is no occurrence of Lymphedema after sentinel lymph node procedure

Answer: c

Explanation: Lymphatic cancer rates are up to 5% for the females who underwent sentinel lymph node procedure and rates are from 10 to 30% for females after axillary lymph node dissection.

Question 167: A patient named Bill Bezos has been experiencing delirium. He is also suffering from marked confusions and hallucinations. Bill believes that the nurse is her daughter and he asks her if everyone at home is alright. The most appropriate reply for the nurse would be?

a) " I am your nurse Mary Lisa".

b) " Please stop dreaming bill".

c) "Yes, everyone is fine back home".

d) "I am not your child'.

Answer: a

Explanation: It would be very helpful for the patient if the nurse tries to orient him by clarifying his name. Delirium is very common for the patients who are at the end of their life.

Question 168: How will the nurse react when the patient says, " I wanted God to help me to cure cancer but I'm worried that he let me get cancer as I was so angry on him?"

a) The nurse offers contact of a social worker to counsel patient

b) The nurse explains that the religion is not a part of the nursing expertise therefore gives the contact of patient's clergy person.

c) The nurse explores patient's feeling of anger and abandonment

d) The nurse offers sleeping pill for the patient so that the patient can rest enough to overcome such thoughts.

Answer: c

Explanation: As a part of spiritual assessment, nurse are advised to explore the feelings of the patient so that the nurse can even more clearly understand about the worries that the patient undergo and can give appropriate solution to make the patient relaxed.

Question 169: Michelle, a patient with breast cancer asks the nurse during counselling, "How long should I wait for my pregnancy after chemotherapy?". The nurse replies by saying,

a) You should wait at least one year

b) No delay is necessary

c) Infertility is said to be the permanent side effect of the therapy

d) Pregnancy will increase the chances of recurrence

Answer: a

Explanation: There is no decrease in the women who gets pregnant after chemotherapy. Therefore, Michelle is recommended to wait one to five years following cessation of all treatment.

Question 170: Harry has been diagnosed with stage IV lung cancer and brain metastasis. He has been receiving whole brain radiation therapy. Which of the following is considered as the intent of the treatment?
a) Palliative
b) Prevention of disease (prophylactic)
c) Curative
d) Boosting immune response (adjuvant)
Answer: a
Explanation: The main purpose of radiation therapy is to reduce the symptoms that are generally caused due to brain metastasis.

Question 171: Among the following condition of the cancer patient, who is most likely to experience sexual dysfunction?
a) A patient and partner who schedule time for their sexual activity.
b) A patient who has a history of marital discord
c) A female patient with hypertension
d) A young and newly married patient
Answer: b
Explanation: Greater risk for sexual difficulties are more likely to be experienced by the patients who were having marital issue in their relationship before the diagnosis of cancer.

Question 172: Janet is newly diagnosed with cancer so she has quit her job and other social activity. What will be the nurse's response to Janet?
a) By asking about the activity she enjoyed the most before starting treatment
b) By asking her to focus on her cancer
c) By encouraging her that she will be able to join after treatment
d) By saying that her friends would be proud of Janet being a brave overcoming cancer
Answer: a
Explanation: Improvement in successful adjustments include discussing her thoughts and feelings safely with an attentive and professional listener. So it is better to make the patient feel stress-free during the entire process.

Question 173: Doxorubicin is given to patient through peripheral IV catheter. The patient reports burning at the site without any swelling. What will be the initial action of the nurse?

a) Administration is continued while observing the site
b) Patient's arm reposition
c) Stop the administration of the drug
d) 10 ml of 0.9% of normal saline is flushed

Answer: c

Explanation: Since Doxorubicin causes damage of tissue, it is advised to stop administrating the drug when there is a report of burns.

Question 174: The actions that require the input source from every individual of the multidisciplinary team is?

a) Improving pain medications
b) Skin care routines
c) Development of care plan
d) Medications for healthy appetite

Answer: c

Explanation: Since the decision making plan is a shared exercise, every member of the multidisciplinary team should be involved in the development of care plan. The individual team members can assume responsibility of specific roles such as stress reduction in which they are involved directly.

Question 175: What action will the nurse take if the family members of the dying patient disagree on placing the feeding tube?

a) Encourages the family to go through similar cases
b) Explains that only the management can make decisions
c) Meets the family to discuss the goals of care
d) Communicates with the social workers to begin the process

Answer: c

Explanation: Generally the family members of a dying patient find it difficult to identify the beneficial care that the patient requires. Therefore it is necessary for the nurse to coordinate the family members and provide support by clarifying doubts, educating family members and providing proper communication with the presence of health care officials.

Question 176: The role of proto oncogene is to ?

a) Causes programmed cell death

b) Promote cell division

c) Stimulate angiogenesis

d) Promote cell division

Answer: B

Explanation: Specialization and division of normal cells are promoted by proto oncogene. The change in genetic sequence can result in uncontrolled cell growth, that results in the formation of tumor. Transfer of proto oncogene to oncogene usually occurs in 3 ways: Point mutation, Translocation and Amplification.

Question 177: Spouse of the patient has been receiving benefits through the Hospice Medicare Benefits. Which of the following is expressed after proper understanding of the teaching?

a) " The coverage of curative chemotherapy will continue for several months"

b) " This benefit can only control the patient's pain"

c)" I will call my hospice provider before taking my spouse to the emergency department"

d) " Curative chemotherapy treatment coverage shall continue for several months"

Answer: c

Explanation: Before calling an ambulance for transporting the patient to the emergency department, family members should be taught to contact their contracted hospice provider.

Question 178: The state of having lost their significant person is generally termed as?

a) Guilt

b) Happiness

c) Grief

d) Bereavement

Answer: d

Explanation: Member who is said to have the closest bond or a legal connection with the deceased person are mostly considered as bereaved.

Question 179: Robert is allowed to participate in phase 2 clinical trial though he doesn't know to speak English. The patient's grandson wishes to translate to receive informed

consent. Which of the following will be the most appropriate option?

a) Having an interpreter to translate with grandson present

b) Allowing grandson to act as an interpreter

c) Language barrier shall disallow patient's participation.

d) Having an interpreter to translate without grandson.

Answer: a

Explanation: It is recommended, a professional interpreter be used to facilitate the process of translating in the presence of his grandson as the member of family could not exactly emote the feeling of Robert.

Question 180: Continuous Quality Improvement, or CQI, is a management philosophy that organizations use to reduce waste, increase efficiency, and increase internal (meaning, employees) and external (meaning, customer) satisfaction. Which among the following is the core concept of CQI?

a) Problems relate to processes and variations in process lead to variations in results

b) Systemic process improvement to be successful

c) Institute organizational transparency

d) Change emanates from the top

Answer: a

Explanation: Core concept of CQI: problems relate to process and variations in process lead to variation in result. Quality and success includes meeting or exceeding internal and external customer's need and expectations. This mainly focusses on 4 step loop process PLAN, DO, CHECK, ACT.

Question 181: What will the next step of the nurse after administering long acting morphine tablet instead of long acting oxycodone?

a) Call the risk management department to guide the documentation

b) Monitoring the patient for next 8 hours continuously

c) Stopping the further medication of patient

d) Notify the patient and the physician of error

Answer: d

Explanation: When any injury occurs to the patient due to the error, it is advised to provide full explanation to the patient and also about the long and short term effects as it is important that the nurse offers a full disclosure of events and what has to be done next.

Question 182: Shortness of breath, fatigue and swelling are reported by the patient who

has been scheduled for chemotherapy. Physical assessment reveals neck vein distention, edema of the hands, tachycardia, and cyanosis. What will be instructed by the nurse to the patient before calling a physician?

a) Lie flat and prepares the patient for thoracotomy

b) Sit up and anticipates an order for a chest-x-ray

c) Lie flat and prepares the patient for echocardiogram

d) Sit up and begins chemotherapy infusion

Answer: b

Explanation: When the blood flow through superior Vena Cava gets compromised, it results in venous congestion proximal to the occlusion and restricted cardiac output. It generally appears as the symptoms for superior Vena Cava syndrome. The chest x-ray is said to be one of the finest methodology to determine this syndrome which shows positive in 80 to 85% cases.

Question 183: Marcus with recurrent cancer is deteriorating due to his old age. His children are not sure of his wishes. Discussion with family and friends helps?

a) To focus on family desire for the patient

b) To find the available and appropriate option

c) To divide the property of the patient equally

d) To agree with the hospital ethics teams

Answer: a

Explanation: A proper communication between the nurse and the family members ensures to gain more information on Marcus's last wishes.

Question 184: 5 mg of immediate release oxycodone is released 5 to 6 times daily when Mr.Smith receives 10mg of Sustained release Oxycodone for every 12 hours. Which of the following order has to be requested for the best adjustment in pain medication regimens?

a) 10 mg of sustained-release oxycodone every 8 hours

b) 30 mg of immediate-release oxycodone every 6 hours

c) 30 mg of sustained-release oxycodone every 12 hours

d) 10 mg of immediate-release oxycodone every 12 hours

Answer: c

Explanation: The duration of analgesia has to be decreased for the given opioid dose. When there is an improvement in analgesia, 25% opioid dosage is increased, for moderate and strong improvement 50% and 100% of the opioid dosage has to be improved respectively.

Question 185: Thrombocytopenia is referred as the decrease in the number of circulating platelets below 100, 000/mm³.What has to be taught to the patient to avoid the risk due to thrombocytopenia?

a) Walking barefoot

b) Having a haircut

c) Using soft bristled toothbrush

d) High fiber food consumption

Answer: a

Explanation: In order to minimize the bleeding the patients are advised to wear shoes during ambulation in order to maintain skin integrity and avoid injury.

Question 186: Ronnie Reacts by displaying maladaptive response for the diagnosis of cancer. This indicates that Ronnie is?

a) Fighting the treatment for his children

b) Lowering his concentration on treatment

c) Feeling abandoned by God

d) Focusing to live in the present moment

Answer: c

Explanation: The most predictive maladaptive response to the illness will be negative religious actions such as pleading the God for forgiveness, Passively deferring decision to God).

Question 187: A Lymphedema patient was reported using reflexology for the affected arm who was seen in the outpatient clinic. What will the nurse enquire?

a) Recommending to use compression sleeve

b) Can u provide me with more information on this technique?

c) Lymphedema will subside over time

d) This method has a promising cure in clinical trials

Answer: B

Explanation: Successful treatment generally building up good rapport, ensuring cultural sensitivity with non-judgmental social and professional environmental. Therefore open communication about the therapy can provide informal support by the nurse to the patient and family members.

Question 188: **The recently developed teaching booklet about immunotherapy was evaluated. It indicates that there is no increase in the group of patient's understanding about immunotherapy in the booklet. Which among the following has been considered as prominent principle?**
a) Verbal teaching increases the learning efficiency
b) Teaching is more effective when it responds to the need identified by the patient
c) The effectiveness of the learning is determined by the teaching methodology
d) Guideline for evaluation is provided depending on teacher's expectation
Answer: b
Explanation: When planning and developing educational material, it is important to consider the patient's physical, psychosocial and emotional needs.

Question 189: **Rihanna has been diagnosed with breast cancer. She has been receiving radiation therapy. She reports to her nurse over her decreased libidos. What will be the appropriate nursing interventions?**
a) Recommend look good feel better programs
b) Gives instructions about the vaginal dilators
c) Explores patient's feeling regarding sexular activity
d) Reassures the patient that it will return
Answer: c
Explanation: There is no harm in receiving the information from Rihanna regarding her sexual history in a non-judgmental and non-threatening manner. This shall help in receiving additional information in order to make a plan.

Question 190: **A patient who is nearing death , was noticed with an audible gurgling during breathing by a nurse. How can the nurse explain the sound to the patient's family members visiting the patient?**
a) " This sound is normal for any patient at this stage"
b) " Due to fluid accumulation, congestion in throat and lungs occur"
c)" He is at his end stage"

d) " These are the side effects of his medications"

Answer: B

Explanation: This condition has to be explained by the nurse in a non-frightening terms. The nurse has to avoid conveying it negatively such as stating about his end stage and also about the side effects. The nurse should not give any false hope saying that the condition is normal during this stage. If the gurgling sound is distressing to the family or if it's severe then medications can be given.

Question 191: **Which of the following should be worn by the nurse as a protective equipment while injecting intravesical mitomycin?**

a) One pair of powdered nitrile glove

b) A Plastic face shield

c) A laboratory gown

d) Shoe covers

Answer: b

Explanation: While administering intra vesicle hazardous drugs, it is advised to wear a plastic face shield to avoid the risk of splashing.

Question 192: **While discussing the ethical principles regarding the side effects of chemotherapy to a staff, the nurse tries to put forth her point saying that positive effects should bring more good effects than the negative effects bringing bad. Which of the following ethical principle is this related?**

a) Justice

b) Non harming or inflicting least harm.

c) Beneficence

d) Autonomy

Answer: b

Explanation: Non harming or inflicting least harm is generally known as Nonmaleficence. This is to ensure least harm in order to bring more benefits. The actual act must be good or morally neutral with more positive benefits though it has negative effects also.

Question 193: **Which among the following is developed as secondary malignancy in patients who have Hodgkin lymphoma?**

a) Ovarian cancer

b) Skin cancer

c) Colorectal cancer

d) Leukemia

Answer: d

Explanation: Some the secondary malignancy for the patient with Hodgkin lymphoma includes Leukemia, myelodysplasia syndromes, non-Hodgkin lymphoma, Breast cancer, lung cancer and thyroid cancer.

Question 194: Among the following option, which is the best mediation to increase the patient's adherence for taking oral chemotherapy at home?

a) In order make the patient take over the counter medicine for nausea

b) It will be easier for the patient to take up the refill when the supply runs out during the next appointment

c) It will be easier to monitor the patient regarding the side effects

d) In order to make the patient feel convenient about taking a double dose in case if the patient missed the medication

Answer: c

Explanation: Monitoring the patient regarding the medication side effects can ensure proper treatment in advance. This can also be a precaution of any other side effects that can be caused due to other medicine with similar composition.

Question 195: Oral mucositis is caused by?

a) Fluorouracil

b) Interleukin 2

c) Paracetamol

d) Amoxicillin

Answer: a

Explanation: By Administering Fluorouracil alone or in combination with other chemotherapy agent can increase the risk of mucositis.

Question 196: Which of the following is most likely to treat opioid related constipation?

a) Mineral oil

b) Bowel stimulants

c) Laxative

d) Tea tree oil

Answer: b

Explanation: Bowel stimulants inhibits propulsive peristalsis. This can be used to treat constipation related to usage of opioids.

Question 197: When the adult children of the patient who passed away approaches the nurse expressing the feelings, then the nurse can provide support to the family by?
 a) Validating these as normal feelings of grief
 b) Encouraging a family conference
 c) Validating the necessity of counseling for these feelings
 d) Encouraging discussion with Physician

Answer: a

Explanation: Family members will grieve for the loss of their loved ones which is normal and expected reaction. Nurses can provide support to the family by validating the normal grief. Normal manifestations of grief include: sadness, anger, guilt, anxiety, loneliness, fatigue, helplessness, yearning, emancipation, relief, and numbness.

Question 198: What will be the duration of nadir to occur, after completing the chemotherapy treatment cycle?
 a) 1- 3 weeks
 b) 2- 5 weeks
 c) 3 weeks
 d) 7- 10 days

Answer: d

Explanation: After completing the complete chemotherapy cycle, nadir occurs within 7- 10 days after chemotherapy.

Question 199: Darbepoetin Alfa has been administered for the patient with advanced stage of breast cancer. Which among the following are the risk associated according to patient's understanding?
 a) Improvement in anemia and the disease may progress
 b) Improvement of anemia causing less risk
 c) Risk are only for those who have large tumors
 d) With each injection the risk of bleeding and infections get doubled.

Answer: a

Explanation: Darbepoetin Alfa injection is used to treat anemia (a lower than normal number of red blood cells). It generally causes progression in causing diseases with a decreased survival rate.

Question 200: **A newly diagnosed patient enquires the nurse about all the tests for clinical staging as suggested by doctor. Which among the following will be the answer given by nurse according to her knowledge regarding staging?**
a) Compares the result across population
b) Assess usual spreading pattern of cancer
c) Evaluates the extend of local and potential metastatic disease
d) Predicts response to treatment
Answer: c
Explanation: Staging is generally done in order to select the appropriate treatment for the cancer depending upon individual patient. It is categorized as pathological, biochemical, clinical and surgical and it's not a direct prediction method.

Question 201: **Harry, Colon cancer survivor wishes to change his job. But he fears that he won't be able to receive his insurance due to his cancer history. What will the nurse advice?**
a) Refer him to a support group
b) Encourages him to speak with a lawyer
c) Inform him about the Americans with Disabilities Act of 1990
d) Provides contact of National Coalition of cancer survivorship.
Answer: c
Explanation: Survivor fears to change job because of loss of insurance. Survivors and their family are protected by ADA act (Americans with Disabilities Act).If insurance coverage is offered to all employees, it must be offered to the cancer survivor or the employer is in violation of the ADA as cancer is considered as disability according to ADA act.

Question 202: **A patient reports of difficulty in doing the regular chores due to dyspnea after completing chemotherapy and radiation therapy for mediastinum. Which of the following is the result of the above symptoms?**
a) Lung Cancer
b) Brain cancer
c) Deconditioning

d) Pneumonitis

Answer: d

Explanation: Dyspnea is said to be a prominent symptom for radiation Pneumonitis. This is because the lung tissue is radiosensitive and generally leads to Pneumonitis after radiation therapy.

Question 203: Robert has reported the following symptoms; a temperature of 102°F (38.7°C), cough, neutrophils count of 200/ mm³ and tenderness around the central venous catheter. What will be the step taken by the nurse?

a) Obtain chest X-ray

b) Initiate colloidal intravenous fluids

c) Obtain blood cultures from 2 sites

d) Administer acetaminophen 500mg.

Answer: c

Explanation: Robert is showing signs of central line bloodstream infection. It shows low neutrophil count. Therefore blood cultures had to be collected before and after administration of antibiotics.

Question 204: The need for descending colostomy has been discussed with John who has Colorectal cancer. What will be the position of stoma?

a) Left lower quadrant

b) Just below the waistline

c) Left upper quadrant

d) Right lower quadrant

Answer: a

Explanation: Descending colostomy location is in the left lower quadrant. Transverse colostomy has its position just below the waist line. Ascending colostomy location is in the right lower quadrant. Sigmoid colostomy is located in left upper quadrant.

Question 205: For which of the following diagnosis, Asparaginase has been demonstrated as a clinical response?

a) Hairy-cell leukemia

b) Acute lymphocytic leukemia

c)Brain cancer

d) Non-small cell cancer

Answer: b

Explanation: Asparaginase often known as L- Asparaginase is used to cure acute lymphoblastic leukemia, acute myeloid leukemia and non Hodgkin lymphoma.

Question 206: Among the following statements made by the patient which of the following options correctly indicate the need of education for prevention of infection?
 a) I won't allow meeting my grandchildren when they are sick.
 b) I do not want to get an influenza shot until all my chemotherapy is finished
 c) I'll be more careful while washing hands after gardening.
 d) I'll keep my wound dressing supplies in a closed container
Answer: b
Explanation: Percentage of the patient achieving protection through influenza vaccine and the risk for adverse effects are very low. The patients and their household contacts must be administered vaccine .NCCN recommends vaccination at least two weeks prior to cytotoxic or immunosuppressive or can be vaccinated during treatment and 3 months after therapy they must be revaccinated.

Question 207: Rochelle, a 34 year old patient has been diagnosed with breast cancer. Counseling has been given to Rochelle and her partner William regarding contraception before chemotherapy. Which of the following statement ensures adequate understanding by the couple?
 a) "Hormone pills are the easiest and the safest method of birth control."
 b) " I don't have to worry about birth control before receiving chemotherapy"
 c)"I will call my gynecologist to discuss about having my tubes tied."
 d) "I will agree to use birth control pills or a reliable barrier method as recommended by my physician."
Answer: d
Explanation: Birth control pills and the barrier methods are suggested by the physician before initiating chemotherapy

Question 208: While providing assistance in resolving patient's spiritual pain during end stage, what will be the prior intervention made by the nurse?
 a) Mobilizing patient's support system
 b) Acknowledge the legitimacy of the patient's pain

c) Encouraging patient to reduce focus on the issues

d) Encouraging reflection of random life events

Answer: b

Explanation: Patients from spiritual and cultural background tend to cause spiritual distress. Encourage verbalization and use family venogram to draw out relationships, fears, hopes and unfinished business will be considered as best acknowledgement of client's spiritual pain.

Question 209: The treatment plan is outlined during initial evaluation and this includes amputation of leg. Suddenly the patients begins to scream and cry saying that he need to walk, play and run with his little children. The response of the nurse will be?

a) The chance of dying is higher if we don't receive amputation.

b) It sounds like you fear your treatment plan, tell me what you know about it

c) The psychiatric nurse will help you cope with the amputation.

d) After fitting with prosthesis, many patients feel better.

Answer: b

Explanation: Nurses can address the underlying feelings with reflective statements that can help patients to gain control and focus on the real issues.

Question 210: A patient receiving a high dosage of methotrexate is administered with intravenous fluid containing sodium bicarbonate. This is done to:

a) Protect against Vomiting

b) Eliminate the leucovorin rescue needs

c)Maintain alkaline urine

d) Reduce sensitivity to reaction

Answer: c

Explanations: Hydrating in order to prevent the renal injury is considered as one of the pretreatment guidelines of methotrexate.

Question 211: William, while recieving chemotherapy has developed tissue swelling in the mouth which increases his mouth pain while brushing with toothpaste. What can be suggested as the alternative brushing method in order to avoid pain?

a) Standard mouthwash

b) Salt water

c) Lidocaine based mouth wash

d) Only water

Answer: b

Explanation: William is advised to use soft bristle tooth brush with salt water. Tooth brush is not advisable for Lidocaine based mouth wash, though it reduces the pain. Normal mouth wash tends to increase irritation. Magic mouth wash or gelclair can be prescribed for better relief in mouth pain.

Question 212: Which antiemetic causes potential side effects such as headache and constipation?

a) Zofran (odansetron)

b) Phenothiazine

c) Aprepitant

d) Amoxicillin

Answer: a

Explanation: Serotonin antibiotics cause side effects such as headache and constipation. Zofran also known as odansetron is one of the serotonin antibiotics. Shivering, muscle rigidity, fever and seizures are other symptoms.

Question 213: Anti Nausea medications are generally administered to the patients to prevent anticipatory nausea due to chemotherapy. Which of the following is said to be the right time to medicate the patient ?

a) Daily during chemotherapy

b) Before Chemotherapy or 2- 3 days after chemotherapy

c) At the time of nausea, during chemotherapy

d) One week before or after chemotherapy

Answer: b

Explanation: As a reaction to chemotherapy, patient may suffer from episodes of nausea and vomiting that causes anticipatory Nausea which can be prevented by giving anti-Nausea medication mostly before Chemotherapy or 2- 3 days after chemotherapy.

Question 214: Before Administering with cyclophosphamide, which among the following medication from the patient's drug profile has to be reported?

a) Celexa

b) Allopurinol

c) Elavil

d) Amoxicillin

Answer: b

Explanation: Allopurinol is a medication used to decrease high blood uric acid levels. Cyclophosphamide is a medication used as chemotherapy and to suppress the immune system. The usage of allopurinol in association with cyclophosphamide can increase the toxicity of the agent especially bone marrow depression by decreasing the renal excretion.

Question 215: What will be the advice of the nurse, when a 64 year old African American patient asks about the prostate screening for her grown sons?

a) An ultrasound guided biopsy of the prostate ate the beginning of age 45

b) A MRI scan at the age of 45

c)A prostate specific antigen test at the age of 45

d) Sulphonyl acid phosphatase at the age of 45

Answer: C

Explanation: According to the American Cancer Society, digital rectal examination and prostate specific antigen testing are considered to be made as the necessary test that has to be taken beginning at the age of 45 for men in concern with the high risk of prostate cancer.

Question 216: A patient's temperature is 39*C and she has tachypnea, tachycardia and leukocytosis (20,000/mm3).She is an immunocompromised patient and she has developed a systematic infection. The infection would be classified as:

a) Multi organ disinfection syndrome

b) Systemic inflammatory response syndrome.

c) Bacteremia.

d) None of the above.

Answer: b

Explanation: Systemic inflammatory response syndrome (SIRS) is a generalized inflammatory response affecting many organ systems. A diagnosis of SIRS is made when two of the following is present: 1. Elevated (>38*C) or subnormal rectal temperature (<36*c). 2. Tachypnea or paCo2<32 mm Hg 3. Tachycardia 4. Leukocytosis (>12,000)orleukopenia(<4000)

Question 217: A patient with permanent colostomy expresses concern of having sexual intercourse. What will the nurse recommend initially?

a) Replace ostomy appliance just before the sexual intercourse

b) Have food before engaging in sexual intercourse

c) Track bowel habits to schedule sexual intercourse

d) Discuss with the therapist before having a sexual intercourse

Answer: c

Explanation: By tracking the expected bowel movements, patient can plan sexual activities easily depending on the bowel habits.

Question 218: **A patient who is undergoing treatment has to be more concerned about intimacy. Which among the following is said to be the most appropriate intervention while discussing this with the patient?**

a) Using PLISSIT model to promote discussion

b) Limiting the discussion to reduce further discomfort

c) Referring all further discussion to the physician

d) Telling the patient to focus only on treatment

Answer: a

Explanation: The nurse generally use PLISSIT Model to promote discussion regarding intimacy and sexuality. The term PLISSIT is an abbreviation for Permission, Limited Information, Specific Suggestion and Intensive Therapy.

Question 219: **Adjuvant chemotherapy is recommended after undergoing surgery for cancer. Here adjuvant chemotherapy is referred to?**

a) Immunotherapy are used to boost body's immune system

b) Drug given to target minimal disease or metastasis

c) Proper investigation of the drugs used along with surgery

d) Treatment are given to the patient who cannot tolerate pain

Answer: b

Explanation: The initial goal of adjuvant therapy is to target any minimal disease or micro metastases for those at risk.

Question 220: **Within a week of chemotherapy a patient with acute lymphoid leukemia experience the following symptoms; Hyperkalemia, Hyperphosphatemia and Hypocalcemia. The above symptoms indicate?**

a) Hyponatremia and hypo-osmolality

b) Septic shock

c) Tumor Lysis Syndrome

d) Consumptive coagulopathy

Answer: c

Explanation: Metabolic abnormalities that are generally associated with tumor lysis syndrome which is an acute lymphocytic leukemia are Hyperkalemia, Hyperphosphatemia and Hypocalcemia.

Question 221: **Despite the use of antiemetics, Megan reports of nausea and vomiting before every chemotherapy. She starts crying and requests to stop the treatment. How will the nurse calms down Megan?**

a) By explaining that everyone experience nausea and Vomiting

b) By suggesting the healthcare provider to stop treatment

c) By discussing integrative therapy options

d) By recommending healthcare provider to reduce dosage

Answer: c

Explanation: Anticipatory nausea can be prevented by integrative or complimentary therapy. These generally include Acupuncture, massage, music therapy etc.

Question 222: **Watson experiences his anger about the diagnosis of cancer as he was about to receive his first chemotherapy. What would be response given by the nurse?**

a) Suggest Watson to participate in treatment plan

b) Asks the physician to delay the treatment

c) Suggest way for the patient to participate in the treatment plan

d) Initiating a referral to social worker

Answer: c

Explanation: Lack the ability to control events that affect life style and goals is perceived as lack of personal goal. The disease and the treatment itself are considered as risk factors. This can be maintained through care and verbalization of feelings.

Question 223: **William who has lung cancer reports of the following symptoms; A sudden acute pleura pain on his left side. He also exhibits dyspnea, Tachypnea, tachycardia, slight cough, and decreased sound in breathing over his left chest. These symptoms are due to?**

a) Myocardial infarction

b) Lymphoma

c) Pneumothorax on left side

d) Acute chest pain

Answer: c

Explanation: The symptoms such as acute pleuritic pain on left side, dyspnea, tachypnea, tachycardia, slight cough are consistent with Pneumothorax on left side. This occurs as a result of erosion of tumor through the surface of the lung. A tension Pneumothorax occurs with tracheal deviation when the air tries to escape. This requires immediate needle decompression and insertion of a chest tube.

Question 224: **The primary purpose of providing multidisciplinary oncology care is to?**

a) Meet the regulatory standards

b) Deliver cost effective services

c) Improvise patient's communication

d) Improve patient's outcome

Answer: d

Explanation: Multidisciplinary oncology care has been identified as a key enabler in the provision of high-quality treatment and care for cancer patients. Multidisciplinary teams aim at improving communication, coordination and decision making between the care professionals.

Question 225: **Which among the following is considered as a true positive indication from cancer screening?**

a) The individual has cancer

b) The individual has a symptom for future diagnosis of cancer

c) The patient doesn't have cancer despite of positive result

d) The patient has cancer despite of the negative result

Answer: a

Explanation: An individual who has cancer shows true positive result during the cancer screening. There are no considerations for the individual with other characteristics.

Question 226: **Aching and throbbing at a particular region is described as?**

a) Neuropathic pain

b) Pain in the internal organ

c) Somatic pain

d) Referred pain

Answer: C

Explanation: Somatic pain occurs when pain receptors in tissues (including the skin, muscles, skeleton, joints, and connective tissues) are activated. Typically, stimuli such as force, temperature, vibration, or swelling activate these receptors.

Question 227: Which of the following action exemplifies safe practice for Robin who has an implanted intrathecal cup for pain management?

a) Arrangements for Robin to have the pump refilling for every 7 months

b) Cleansing the lock port with sanitizer before each use

c) Tracing the path of tube from the patient to pump

d) Special tubes with injection ports

Answer: c

Explanation: An intrathecal pump is a medical device used to deliver medications directly into the space between the spinal cord and the protective sheath surrounding the spinal cord. Tracing the path of line from patient to pump ensures that there is no issue with the pump functionality.

Question 228: Watson expresses his willingness to return back to work after treatment. But sometimes he reports of feeling fatigue. Which among the following is considered as the suitable step for his problem?

a) Discussing with his officials regarding flexible work time.

b) Avoiding discussion with his co-workers who are sick

c) Having a break for a 2 years before commencing work schedule

d) Asking the family member to work and continue with household chores.

Answer: A

Explanation: Watson can probably balance his treatment with work schedules only if he is able to discuss his working hours with his officials and co-workers. Only with reduced work schedules and support from his work environment can facilitate smooth transition to workforce after treatment.

Question 229: Clara, a 20 year old childhood brain cancer survivor is complaining about her sudden weight gain, weakness in muscles, dysmenorrhea and depression. At the age of 5, she underwent radiation therapy and surgery as treatment for cancer. The above

symptoms are the later effects of?

a) Resurgence of Cancer

b) Cardiomyopathy

c) Lack of healthy red blood cells

d) Hypothyroidism

Answer: d

Explanation: Exposure of head and neck to radiation results in Hypothyroidism. This occurs when the thyroid produces insufficient amount of thyroid hormone. Risk increases with increased radiation dosage and for females. Symptoms generally include chronic fatigue, menstrual disturbances, hoarseness in voice, low pulse rate rate, thinning of hair and thickening of skin. It also causes some dementia with hypothyroidism.

Question 230: What is reason for administering whole breast radiation following Lumpectomy for a patient with stage 1 breast cancer?

a) To remove microscopic disease

b) To remove nodal disease

c) To reduce communicable disease

d) To decrease locally advanced disease

Answer: a

Explanation: Radiation therapy is provided after surgery in order to destroy the gross or microscopic disease with a goal of preventing recurrence of tumor.

Question 231: What will be the most appropriate test that the nurse suggest when Ricard's adolescent son approaches for screening?

a) Colonoscopy

b) CA 19-9 test

c) Prostate-specific antigen test

d) Testicular self-examination

Answer: d

Explanation: At the beginning as a teenager, Richard's son must be taught with the testicular self-examination which is considered as the most important prevention method in order to make him aware about the risk factors.

Question 232: Merlin is a foreign born women with breast cancer. She has a lower survival rate when compared to other women with breast cancer who were born in the United States. Which among the following is more likely to attribute to Merlin's condition?

a) Histologic grades of the tumor
b) Differences in the protocol of treatment
c) Access to mammographic treatment
d) Country from where the women have been immigrated.

Answer: c

Explanation: Women like Merlin who are living in other countries don't get easy access to the screening and care for obtaining recommended treatment, which can most likely lead to later stage diagnosis with decreased survival rate.

Question 233: The most prominent symptom of oral mucositis is?

a) Bleeding
b) Eye Infection
c) Pain
d) Headache

Answer: c

Explanation: The common symptom of oral mucositis is pain. Other symptoms include Red, shiny or swollen mouth and gums, Blood in the mouth, Sores in the mouth or on the gums or tongue, Soreness or pain in the mouth or throat, Difficulty swallowing or talking.

Question 234: A patient with breast cancer reports of exhaustion after 3 months of chemotherapy and radiation. How will the nurse respond?

a) Explains the importance of sleep
b) " Physician will suggest antidepressants"
c) Explains that the side effects shall reduce very soon
d) Asks the patient to express the ways it affects the daily routine

Answer: d

Explanation: Usually there is an increase in fatigue that tends to persist for many months in case of multimodal treatment. Therefore assessing the occurrence of chronic fatigue is said to be one important task for the nurse.

Question 235: Focus is made on palliative care for the patient and family in order to:

a) Treat every patient equally in order to meet his / her needs, expectations and cultural beliefs

b) Attend the need of those who love and care for the dying person

c) Provide relief from suffering during the last 6 months of life expectancy

d) Preserve the patient life that is based solely on Clinical technology and scientific advances

Answer: b

Explanation: Palliative care is given to the patient and family in attend the need of those who love and care for the dying person and survivors are provided with bereavement resources following the patient's death.

Question 236: During her childhood, Rosie has received Carmustine. Now, being a 24 year old adult she reports of persistent cough and shortness in breath. Which of the following has high risk of development?

a) Lung embolism

b) Pulmonary Fibrosis

c) Accumulation of pus in pleural space

d) Allergic reaction to the fungus

Answer: b

Explanation: Carmustine also known as bis-chloroethylnitrosourea, BCNU, BiCNU is a medication used mainly for chemotherapy. It is a nitrogen mustard Î²-chloro-nitrosourea compound used as an alkylating agent. It generally causes pulmonary fibrosis.

Question 237: Juliette has stage III C ovarian cancer. After receiving her first line therapy, she became worst again after a little improvement. She demonstrates an understanding of her condition by stating that,

a) " I think I must be overdoing it a bit"

b) " These symptoms are due to chemotherapy"

c)" I'm happy that I won't be needing any additional treatment"

d) " Are clinical trials available for other recurrent disease?"

Answer: d

Explanation: Many patients after receiving their chemotherapy treatment for their stage III c ovarian cancer are reported getting worse after receiving the first line therapy. In case of recurrence of ovarian cancer, clinical trial is known to be the appropriate measure and it should be explored.

Question 238: While developing cancer therapies, it is important to have an understanding about the immunology because:

a) It shows how free radicals are removed from the body

b) It identifies how T cells, B cells and natural killer cells work

c) It assumes the duration of treatment tolerance

d) It creates an impact on treatment choices to maintain the bone marrow function

Answer: b

Explanation: The importance of having an understanding of immunology while developing cancer therapy is to identify how T cells, B cells and natural killer cells work.

Question 239: An 85 years old patient was advised for a surgery and chemotherapy by his physician. But his family members were not convinced with the physician's decision. They advocate palliative care. What will be the response from the nurse when asked by the patient?

a) Assess the patient's values and basis for his preference.

b) Consults hospital ethics committee

c) Helps the patient in completing advanced directives

d) Supports and documents family's preference

Answer: a

Explanation: Thorough assessment has to be made for the decisions involving psychological factors. This includes understanding situations, emotional distress and presence of risk factors.

Question 240: How does the alkylating agent exert their pressure?

a) By disrupting folate dependent metabolic process essential for cell replication

b) By attaching to CD52 on the surface of B and T cells that generally result in antibody dependent lysis.

c) By binding to the DNA strand which prevents DNA replication and cell division

d) By causing the release of toxic free radicals inside the cell and triggering their apoptosis.

Answer: c

Explanation: Alkylating agent generally binds with the DNA strand, breaks the DNA helix strand and interferes with DNA replication. It also prevents the occurrence of cell division.

Question 241: Which of the following has to be administered as initial treatment for the patient with septic shock?

a) IV antifungals

b) Corticosteroids at high dosage

c) IV antibiotics

d) Vasopressors

Answer: c

Explanation: In order to maintain blood pressure and tissue perfusion, the antibiotic therapy generally based on the site of infection and most likely a causative pathogen.

Question 242: A cancer survivor is applying for a job interview. Which among the following should be done by the applicant during the initial interview?

a) The applicant has to explain about the personal qualifications for the job

b) The applicant has to provide medical information and current status

c) The applicant has to contact the interviewer

d) The applicant should not provide details about his cancer treatment

Answer: a

Explanation: Any applicant has to outline only about the job qualifications and requirements. The medical history should not be discussed till the job is offered. All the information regarding the insurance for future treatments and other enquiries has to be made only when their offer is confirmed. Only on any requirement, they can provide information about their cancer history and details.

Question 243: Michelle has metastatic breast cancer. She experiences pain at the site of metastasis during the initiation of tamoxifen. Which among the following clearly explains the pain?

a) Due to progression of disease

b) Due to improper sleeping position

c) A Psychosomatic reaction due to the diagnosis of metastasis

d) A common temporary reaction to the initiation therapy

Answer: d

Explanation: The pain caused during the infusion of tamoxifen is due to tumor flare. The pain lasts only for a short duration and usually disappears with continuous therapy.

Question 244: To whom is the nurse responsible to according to ANA code of ethics?

a) Physician

b) Medical Council

c) Patient

d) Herself

Answer: c

Explanation: Nurse has to ensure the privacy, safety, rights and confidentiality of patient details with respect and care by considering the environment of patients, articulate values and maintenance of professional integrity.

Question 245: A patient named Michael Smith is seen shaking and distraught when the nurse enters his room. Michael has just spoken with his doctor. After seeing the patient's condition the nurse's response should be:

a) Everything will be alright, don't worry.

b) Can I get something for you?

c) Shall I contact your family?

d) You seem worried and shaken, are you alright?

Answer: d

Explanation: The option d is right here because this response allows the patient to understand that the nurse acknowledges his situation .It also allows the patient to discuss his situation with the nurse if he wishes to .The other options do not present this opportunity to the patient.

Question 246: Which of the following intervention is suggested to the patient who has dry desquamation?

a) Hydrogel dressing

b) Aloe Vera dressing

c) Moisturizing skin cream

d) Silver sulphadiazine

Answer: c

Explanation: Skin peeling can have causes that aren't due to underlying disease. Examples include sunburn, grass burn, prolonged time in water or prolonged skin contact with noxious liquid. Moisturizing skin cream can reduce dry desquamation.

Question 247: Why is it important to assess attitudes about illness and care-seeking in a

patient from different racial and ethnic groups?
a) To determine ineffective intervention
b) Tailor treatment approaches to individual patient
c) To effectively change attitudes.
d) To identify socio economic status of the patient.

Answer: b

Explanation: To understand and assist diverse cultural groups with their nursing and health care needs is the aim of transcultural nursing. Assessing the cultural aspects of an individual's lifestyle, health beliefs, and health practices will enhance the nurse's decision making and judgment while providing care to the individual.

Question 248: **The work of epidermal growth factor receptor inhibitors inside the cell is to**
a) Block the binding on the intracellular portion of the receptor
b) Promote the proliferation of non-malignant cells to repair
c) Produce antibodies in recognizing and destroying cancer cells
d) Activate the T cells to mount an immune system attack on cancer cells

Answer: a

Explanation: Epidermal growth factor inhibitors or the protein kinase inhibitors are small molecules that work by blocking the binding site on the intracellular portion of a receptor.

Question 249: **Regina's pain was under control after administering morphine sulfate but due to other side effects she was administered with equianalgesic drug. At what range should the dosage of new drug be initiated?**
a) 25- 50% below equianalgesic drug
b) 25- 50% above the equianalgesic drug
c) 5% below equianalgesic drug
d) 20% above equianalgesic drug

Answer: b

Explanation: When significant side effects occur after providing good relief for the pain, the dose of opioids has to be increased from 25% to 50% below the equianalgesic dose in the situation where cross tolerant symptoms occurs. The opioids has to be turned around the equianalgesic dose if the pain control was not adequate and side effects occurred significantly.

Question 250: Robert has pulmonary metastasis and has been receiving repeated thoracentesis. Which among the following development will the nurse be more concerned about?
a) lung expansion minimization (trapped lung)
b) Lung embolism
c) Constriction of airways in the lung
d) Pneumonitis
Answer: a
Explanation: Development of unexpanded lung or trapped lung is the cause of repeated thoracentesis.

Question 251: A cancer patient reports of following symptoms; appearance of white lesions on the tongue and inside of her cheeks, the tissues is irritated painful with slight bleeding. Which among the following is the best treatment?
a) Ampicillin
b) Caphosol
c) Mouth wash with lemon swabs
d) Nystatin an antifungal medication for oral suppression
Answer: d
Explanation: These are very common in cancer patients and occurs due to oral candidiasis. To treat and relieve this condition, nystatin oral suspension is used. If there is no cure of candidiasis then diflucan can be prescribed. During the night and after the meals dentures should be removed for cleansing. Tongue appears reddened causing irritation with disappearance of white lesions in some cases.

Question 252: A patient is treated with posaconazole. Which of the following side effects should be informed to the patient regarding the treatment?
a) Pancreatitis
b) Torsades de Pointes
c) Anemia
d) Bone marrow aplasia
Answer: b
Explanation: Torsades de pointes is a specific form of polymorphic ventricular tachycardia in patients with a long QT interval. This also include few other life threatening reactions

such as hepatocellular damage and allergic reactions

Question 253: The formal closure activities that should be done once the patient dies are:
a) Helping the family in making funeral rituals.
b) Establishing an ongoing long relationship.
c) Sending a condolence card.
d) All of the above.

Answer: c

Explanation: Sending a condolence card is the most appropriate answer here as it might help them find closure and the other options here are outside the expected responsibilities of a nurse.

Question 254: Rochelle has been diagnosed with breast cancer and she is 14 weeks pregnant. She is more concerned about the treatment effects on her baby. Which among the following information does the nurse provide?
a) Occurrence of spontaneous abortion
b) Decrease in doses to ensure safety
c) About the initiation of chemotherapy after pregnancy
d) Minimal effects of chemotherapy after first trimester

Answer: d

Explanation: Chemotherapy can be safely administered after first trimester. This is because the baby's organs are said to develop during 12 to 14 weeks of pregnancy. Therefore chemotherapy possess less risk to the fetus.

Question 255: When developing an education program which of the following action must be performed first?
a) Determine educational objective
b) Formulating criteria for evaluation
c) Assess learning needs
d) Educational methods had to be selected

Answer: c

Explanation: When a nurse develops an educational program ,the key point to be noted is to assess learning requirements. This is the categorized as the first step in determining educational objectives, selecting educational methods, and later formulates criteria for evaluation.

Question 256: Which of the following terminology is associated with the malignant tumor originating in the epithelial cells?
a) Adeno and squamous
b) Osteo and Condra
c) Lympho and Myelo
d) Lipo and Condra
Answer: a
Explanation: Tumour classification is done by the origin of tissue. Squamous cell, adenocarcinoma, basal cells and choriocarcinoma are the malignant tumour arising from the epithelium.

Question 257: Which among the following is an example for adaptive or specific immunity?
a) Large lymphocyte production
b) Cell mediated response
c) Inflammatory response
d) Acute phase protein production
Answer: b
Explanation: Cell mediated immunity doesn't involve antibodies and they are mediated by the T cells and their cytokine products.

Question 258: A patient has a platelet count of 15000/ mm³. Which of following intervention should the nurse institute while attending the patient?
a) Providing massage to reduce the pain
b) Placing warm hot bags on the injected region
c) Using mouth swabs to complete oral care
d) Obtaining blood samples through large needles
Answer: c
Explanation: Sponges and bristle less toothbrush are used for the patient who has platelets counts less than 20,000/ mm³. Therefore it is advised to complete the oral care with mouth swabs.

Question 259: Richard reports of certain symptoms after receiving a high dose of external beam radiation for lung cancer 8 weeks ago. This symptoms include development of dyspnea and non productive cough. In the area of his previous radiation treatment, a chest x-ray shows open ground glass opacification. Which among the following is the result of the above symptoms?

a) Radiation pneumonitis
b) Increased libidos
c) Bilateral atelectasis
d) Cardiac tamponade

Answer: a

Explanation: For about 15% patients receiving high dose of external beam radiation can cause radiation pneumonitis. With increased dyspnea and non productive cough, this can be characterized. Other symptoms include occurrence of blood while coughing(hemoptysis) in several places. The symptoms are evident on radiographs through ground glass opacification. This symptoms generally occur during the second or third month of the therapy. At certain cases, respiratory failure occurs.

Question 260: A nurse has been assigned to take care of 5 patients. She provides documentation and assessment for only 4 patients as she had misread the entire agreement. The legal principle that applies to this situation is?

a) Non harming
b) Breach of duty
c) Dereliction of duty
d) Testimonial proof

Answer: b

Explanation: A breach of the duty of care occurs when one fails to fulfill his or her duty of care to act reasonably in some aspect.

Question 261: Among the following, the early symptoms for increased intracranial pressure is related to?

a) Confusion
b) Nausea
c) Fatigue

d) Decortication

Answer: a

Explanation: Increased intracranial pressure shows symptoms such as restlessness and confusion.

Question 262: Bob is said to have frequent seizure despite of receiving hospice service for brain tumor. He was not able tolerate oral Anticonvulsants as he has only limited days for survival. What will be the nurse's anticipation?

a) Keppra

b) Liquid lorazepam

c) Fentanyl patch

d) Phenothiazine

Answer: b

Explanation: Liquid lorazepam is used to treat anxiety. Lorazepam belongs to a class of drugs known as benzodiazepines which act on the brain and nerves (central nervous system) to produce a calming effect. This drug works by enhancing the effects of a certain natural chemical in the body.

Question 263: Which of the following medications requires mandatory enrollment in a program to ensure teaching about risks to a fetus is provided?

a) Capecitabine

b) Sorafenib

c) Lenalidomide

d) Everolimus

Answer: c

Explanation: Lenalidomide is only available under the REVAssist® program to ensure patients are properly informed of fetal risks.

Question 264: What is the long term complication for the patient who is receiving hormonal therapy for prostate cancer?

a) Cardiac dysfunction

b) Lymphedema

c) Adverse skeletal events

d) Ulcers

Answer: c

Explanation: Skeletal-related events (SREs) are a common complication of bone metastases, and have serious negative consequences for patients with castrate-resistant prostate cancer (CRPC). Bone mineral loss and decreased testosterone from hormonal agents cause adverse skeletal events.

Question 265: Merlin, a cancer patient has lost four pounds since the beginning of her Chemotherapy-treatment. What will be first reaction of the nurse after finding it during her home visit?

a) Asks Merlin to consult physician

b) Suggests high-protein and high calorie-food

c) Investigates the reason for weight loss

d) Arrange for meals on the wheels service

Answer: c

Explanation: There are several factors that affect weight of individual during chemotherapy. Therefore it is advisable to learn about the cause of weight loss from the patient through the heath care team.

Question 266: Robin has been diagnosed with lung cancer and admitted in the hospital. He will be discharged after he gets administered with cisplatin and etoposide. What are the information that are included in the discharge report?

a) Careful observation of urine for the next two days for blood and immediately report its presence.

b) Development of hiccups are considered as normal

c) A fever should be reported immediately to the physician

d) Ringing in the ear continues to increase due to etoposide

Answer: c

Explanation: Follow up care and symptom management are some of the primary understanding of the patient after the pre chemotherapeutic teaching. The risks factors and the symptoms are more important notes to be informed to the patient.

Question 267: William was diagnosed with acute myeloid leukemia. He reported of bleeding gums and refracts to random donor platelets. Which among the following has to be anticipated initially?

a) Obtaining a type and crosshatching for cryoprecipitate

b) CMV-negative platelets can be transfused

c) Administer human leukocyte antigen-matched platelets

d) Fresh frozen plasma can be administered

Answer: c

Explanation: In order to inhibit refraction to random donor platelets and bleeding of gums the patient must be administered initially with human leukocyte antigen matched platelets.

Question 268: Richard has completed treatment for neck and head cancer. He is at high risk for which secondary malignancy?

a) Kidney cancer

b) Bile duct cancer

c) Lung cancer

d) Glioblastoma multiforme

Answer: c

Explanation: Lung cancer or Buccal cancer are said to cause higher risk of secondary malignancy affecting the skin and mucosa after completing the treatment for neck and head cancer.

Question 269: Patient who has been undergoing treatment for cancer fails to respond to the treatment. When this has been informed to the patient, what will be the initial nursing interventions?

a) Asks the patient to share the feelings after hearing the news

b) Providing time for self processing by the patient

c) Asking family members to provide verbal support

d) Reviewing the treatment possibilities as referred by the physician

Answer: a

Explanation: The nurse should be more responsible about the patient's feeling after hearing about the failure of treatment rather than reviewing the treatment possibility as prescribed by the physician.

Question 270: From which among the following does the squamous cell carcinoma of esophagus tends to arise?

a) Abdominal esophagus

b) Proximal esophagus

c) Lymph

d) Hyaline cartilage

Answer: b

Explanation: Squamous cell carcinoma (SCC) is an invasive epithelial malignancy that arises from the prickle-squamous cell layers of the epidermis and shows differentiation of keratinocytes. The squamous cell carcinoma tends to arise from the proximal esophagus.

Question 271: There is a significant increase in the risk of developing a breast cancer. Which among the following people has a higher chance of risk?
a) Menarche at age 13
b) First pregnancy at age of 31
c) Mother diagnosed before 60 years of age
d) Menopause at the age of 53

Answer: c

Explanation: Age appears to be a major factor in determining the risk of a patient regarding breast cancer. A mother who has been diagnosed with breast cancer at the age of 60 years of age is said to be facing a risk 2 to 4 times higher than that of those without these risk factors.

Question 272: Pathological process of syndrome of inappropriate anti-diuretic hormone include?
a) Decreased sodium secretion by kidneys.
b) Urine osmolality is less than serum osmolality
c) Increased serum sodium concentration
d) Increased reabsorption of water by the renal tubules

Answer: d

Explanation: Renal tubules increase the reabsorption of water causing increased urine osmolarity is said to be the primary characteristic occurrence of symptom of inappropriate anti-diuretic hormone.

Question 273: Which of the following side effects has an increased risk for the patient who is receiving Bevacizumab exhibiting proteinuria?
a) Mucositis
b) Cardiac dysfunction

c) Hypertension

d) Peripheral neuropathy

Answer: C

Explanation: Proteinuria is caused by relatively benign (non-cancerous) or temporary medical conditions. These include dehydration, inflammation and low blood pressure. Intense exercise or activity, emotional stress, aspirin therapy and exposure to cold can also trigger proteinuria. Bevacizumab can result in hypertension.

Question 274: **Clara is a premenopausal patient who has been diagnosed with cancer. After the treatment, when can Clara expect her menstruation again?**

a) After 6 months

b) After 3 months

c) After 2 years

d) After a year

Answer: b

Explanation: If Clara doesn't get her menses within 3 months after her treatment, then she is most likely to have a permanent ovary failure.

Question 275: **How does filgrastim maintains the dose intensity of the treatment regimen?**

a) By reducing the risk of damaging the heart muscle

b) By reducing the occurrence of Nausea

c) By reducing the febrile neutropenia occurrence

d) By saving the body from the attack of toxic substance (Leucovorin rescue).

Answer: c

Explanation: Filgrastim under the name of neupogen is a medication used to treat low neutrophil count. It is used to increase white blood cells for gathering during leukapheresis. It is used to reduce the risk of fibrils neutropenia.

Question 276: **William, a cancer patient plans of going through a clinical trial that compares current standard treatment with a chemotherapeutic agent. Which among the following denotes the exact phase of this trial?**

a) 5

b) 7

c) 3

d) 2

Answer: c

Explanation: Phase 3 trials are conducted to confirm and expand on safety and effectiveness results from Phase 1 and 2 trials, to compare the drug to standard therapies for the disease or condition being studied, and to evaluate the overall risks and benefits of the drug. Phase 3 clinical trials have a primary goal of establishing efficacy and comparing with the current standard.

Question 277: Among the following, who has increased risk of developing a graft-versus-host disease?

a) A 30-years- old patient received an autologous hematopoietic stem cells transfer

b) A 60-years-old patient received an allogeneic transplant from a unrelated donor.

c) A 25-years-old patient received a tandem autologous stem cell transplant

d) A 42-years- old patient received a syngeneic hematopoietic stem cell transplant

Answer: b

Explanation: Patients above the age of 60 years are at higher risk of graft-versus-host disease. This is because they had undergone an allogeneic transplant from a matched and unrelated donor.

Question 278: Michael, a 25 year old patient has been diagnosed with cancer. Physician prescribed him with temozolomide. What will be the initial instruction given to the patient?

a) Medication must be taken at bedtime on an empty stomach

b) Ingestion of medicine with full glass of milk

c) Medication must be taken after dinner

d) Always consume a magnesium supplement

Answer: a

Explanation: In order to decrease the risk of nausea and vomiting, it is advised to take temozolomide on an empty stomach.

Question 279: After hematopoietic stem cell transplant, Robert was taught about the discharge medication. Which among the following explains the purpose of tacrolimus?

a) It helps to prevent fungal pneumonia

b) It avoids sinusoidal obstruction syndrome

c) It prevents graft-versus-host disease

d) It prevents Nausea and vomiting sensation

Answer: c

Explanation: Tacrolimus also known as protopoc and profag, is an immunosuppressive drug that is generally administered to a Robert after allogeneic organ transplant. This generally helps in lowering the risk of organ rejection.

Question 280: David is 70 year old having prostate cancer and vertebral tenderness . He bears so much pain during his bowel movements. He also suffering with muscle loss and sensory paresthesia. The appropriate cause for this is:

a) urinary infection

b) spinal cord compression

c) Lower Back strain

d) loss of urine or bowel control

Answer: b

Explanation: Condition of spinal cord compression occurs as tumors invade epidural space of spinal cord. Symptoms include back pain ,muscle loss, reduced bladder function and vertebral tiredness. Fast growing tumor are treated with surgery and others with radiation.

Question 281: Which of the following has the possibility to occur as secondary malignancy for Rochelle who has ovarian cancer?

a) Hodgkin carcinoma

b) Ocular Melanoma

c) Leiomyosarcoma

d) Gastric carcinoma

Answer: b

Explanation: Rochelle has a high risk of developing an eye cancer as a secondary malignancy.

Question 282: Among the following, which is termed as the shortest phase of the cell cycle?

a) Meiosis

b) Prophase

c) Gap 1

d) Mitosis

Answer: d

Explanation: Anaphase is the shortest phase of mitosis. In anaphase, the sister chromatids are pulled apart to opposite ends of the cell.

Question 283: Which among the following statements indicate the need for additional teaching regarding the coverage provided by the Family Medical Leave Act?
a) " I know I'm eligible because I'm an American citizen"
b) " I can take up to 15 weeks of leave "
c)" It helps me to take good care of my sister who is also a cancer patient "
d) " It is difficult because my time off is unpaid "

Answer: a

Explanation: The Family and Medical Leave Act of 1993 is a United States labor law requiring covered employers to provide employees with job-protected and unpaid leave for qualified medical and family reasons. It provides unpaid leave to care for the family member who is seriously affected due to cancer.

Question 284: A patient is suddenly diagnosed with surgical unresectable renal cell carcinoma that has suddenly metastasized to Liver. Which of the following biological therapy has to be prescribed?
a) Intravenous drug temsirolimus
b) Adrucil (flurouracil)
c) epidermal growth factor receptor (EGFR) inhibitor (Cetuximab)
d) Nilotinib

Answer: a

Explanation: Among the 30 percent of the individual during renal cell carcinoma experience metastasis. During those periods biological therapy such as temsirolimus is suggested instead of chemotherapy.

Question 285: Which among the following technique supports the healthy communication pattern between the patient and nurse?
a) After providing all the information, the questions has to be limited.
b) The objective and factual information has to be provided regarding the treatment plan
c) Physical distance has to be established between the parties

d) Feedbacks has to be obtained regarding the preferences and experiences

Answer: d

Explanation: Healthy communication can be established when the nurse is able to obtain information from the patient regarding the treatment process, understanding of the concepts and reaction to the treatment. This can promote more open and honest conversation between the patient and the nurse.

Question 286: A patient after first chemotherapy experiences chemotherapy induced alopecia. Which among the following indicates the time frame of alopecia?
a) After 1 month
b) After 2 month
c) Before 24 hours
d) After 2 weeks

Answer: d

Explanation: Chemotherapy induced alopecia generally referred to the hair loss that the patient experience after initial treatment. The patient experience hair loss 2 weeks post initial chemotherapy.

Question 287: Which of the following cancer is associated with a patient exposed to radon for a longer duration?
a) Bladder Cancer
b) Colorectal / Bowel Cancer
c) Lung Cancer
d) Breast Cancer

Answer: c

Explanation: Studies and researches confirm that there is a connection between the radon exposure and Lung Cancer. But there is no such studies confirming the link between breast bowel and bladder cancer with radon exposure.

Question 288: In order to reduce the noise rattled breathing for a dying patient which of the following non pharmacological interventions is suitable?
a) Humidifying oxygen
b) Executing nasopharyngeal suctions
c) Increasing the morphine infusion rate
d) Relocating/Repositioning to clear secretion

Answer: d

Explanation: Repositioning in order to clear secretion can reduce the noise and rattled breathing caused by the dying patient.

Question 289: The highest incident and mortality of prostate is reported among which of the following groups in United States of America?
a) Hispanic Americans
b) Asian Americans
c) Non Hispanic Caucasian
d) African Americans

Answer: d

Explanation: African American males are said to have the highest mortality rate for prostate cancer which is twice that of Caucasian males in United States.

Question 290: Which among the following measures provides relief for the patient who has had persistent nausea and vomiting despite of receiving medication for controlling the symptoms?
a) By laying flat on the floor
b) By avoiding dinner
c) By taking a deep breath and having control of swallowing manners
d) By in taking large volume of fluid

Answer: c

Explanation: The vomit reflex of the patient can be avoided by having a deep breath and with controlled swallowing. The fluids should not be taken in large volume. Instead should be sipped in small amounts throughout the day.

Question 291: A common and preventable cause of anxiety in Robin who is suffering from cancer is?
a) Disturbances in sleep
b) Uncontrolled pain
c) Changes in the treatment protocol
d) Spiritual distress

Answer: b

Explanation: Chronic and poorly controlled pain can eventually lead to anxeity and depression. This can be controlled by having medication to suppress the pain caused due to the cancer treatment.

Question 292: While getting Doxorubicin infused Mike reports Pruritus above the peripheral IV site. The nurse observes a redness along the vein with a brisk sustained blood return. Which among the following reactions does the above symptoms indicate?
a) An Extravasation
b) Flare reaction
c) Radiation recall
d) Psychosomatic response
Answer: b
Explanation: Flare reaction or the local allergic reactions are caused by the drugs that are irritants. These reactions are very common during chemotherapy. This also causes symptoms such as itching, blotchiness or streaking along or next to the vein receiving the infusion. It generally occurs without the presence of swelling or pain.

Question 293: Occurrence of nausea is generally due to cancer or due to the treatment of cancer. Patient are taught with some basic self-care strategies that encourages patients to ?
a) Eat food that are cold at room temperature
b) High protein and potassium rich food
c) Avoid brushing after nauseating
d) Consume sauces and gravies
Answer: a
Explanation: In addition to pharmacological management, patient are given self-care treatments such as eating food that are cold at room temperature as the aroma of hot food increases nausea.

Question 294: Clara has been diagnosed with stage 3 cervical cancer. There are certain situations in which she may defer discussions about alteration in body image and sexual intimacy prior to the cancer treatment. Which among the following is likely to match the above reasons?
a) Depersonalization of the disease experience
b) Expectations of unrealistic outcomes
c) Concerned of being perceived as vain.
d) Expectation of experiencing minimal symptom for treatment

Answer: C

Explanation: Sometimes while having a discussion with her partner about sexuality Clara seems to feel like being in vain, as she feels that the discussion seems to inappropriate and can embarrass when compared to the seriousness of her treatment.

Question 295: **What is duration within which manifestation of the symptoms for anaphylactic reaction occur?**
 a) 60 minutes
 b) 45 minutes
 c) 30 minutes
 d) 20 minutes

Answer: c

Explanation: Manifestation of the symptoms for anaphylactic reaction generally occurs within 30 minutes of initial administration of the medication.

Question 296: **The protective equipment that is recommended during the clean-up of the hazardous medical spill is**
 a) Cloth gown
 b) Face shield
 c) Vinyl surgical gloves
 d) Latex gloves

Answer: b

Explanation: Whenever the hazardous medication are realized into the environment due to any spill, face shield will provide proper protection from any sudden splash causing damage to the eyes and face while cleaning the spill.

Question 297: **A patient with renal carcinoma has been administered with sunitinib. Patient reports of burning sensation, tingling and redness in the palm and foot while receiving sunitinib. Which among the following is the result of the above symptoms?**
 a) Acneiform rash
 b) Erythema multiform major
 c) Darkened patches and spots on skin
 d) Palmar plantar erythrodysesthesia

Answer: d

Explanation: Hand-foot syndrome is also called palmar-plantar erythrodysesthesia. It is a side effect of some cancer treatments. Hand-foot syndrome causes redness, swelling, and pain on the palms of the hands or on the soles of the feet. Sometimes blisters also appear.

Question 298: William has been newly diagnosed with Hodgkin lymphoma. Through the following clinical diagnosis, William is determined to have an unfavorable prognosis?

a) Involvement of several lymph nodes

b) Absolute lymphocyte count 400/ mm³

c) Hemoglobin 15g/dl

d) Thrombocytopenia

Answer: b

Explanation: Hodgkin lymphoma is a cancer of the lymphatic system. An absolute lymphocyte count of less than 600/mm3 is an unfavorable prognostic finding for a patient with advanced Hodgkin lymphoma.

Question 299: The required premedication causes drowsiness. The nurse informs the patient about the drowsiness that occurs due to medication. Therefore the patient request the nurse for delaying the treatment so that patient performs the prayer during sunset. The nurse should first

a) Require that a waiver be signed to delay treatment

b) Delay the treatment for 24 hours

c) Assess to determine if a delay is permissible

d) Informing the patient that the treatment can't be delayed

Answer: C

Explanation: The nurses should support only spiritual and cultural practices that are non-harming to patient's health

Question 300: William reports difficulty in manipulating a toothbrush and silverware before administering fourth dose of cisplatin. Which among the following is said to be the initial intervention?

a) Arranging an occupational therapy consultation.

b) Document the findings and reporting to the physician

c) Instructing the patient to take seek attention regarding meals and oral hygiene

d) Assuring patient that these are temporary side effects of chemotherapy

Answer: D

Explanation: Cisplatin is among the platinum based chemotherapy drug that is most powerful and widely used against cancer. This generally causes trouble in walking, numbness and pain with start and continue proximally.

Question 301. A 41-year-old women is diagnosed to be suffering from stage IV ovarian cancer. She requests to consult a different doctor because she believes that her doctor has misdiagnosed her. Which stage of Elizabeth Kubler-Ross's stages of grief is she currently suffering from?
 a) Denial
 b) Bargaining
 c) Anger
 d) Betrayal
Answer: b
Explanation: The patient is currently in the stages of bargaining; in this stage the patient might try to change one or multiple doctors in a bid to change the outcome of the result. Bargaining is one of the five stages of grief, the other stages are namely denial, anger, depression and acceptance.

Thank you for purchasing this book!

I know you could have picked any number of books to read, but you picked this book and for that I am extremely grateful.

What Do You Think of this OCN Exam Practise Questions Book?

I hope that this book added value and quality to your life and helped you in your OCN Exam preparation. If you liked this book and found some benefit in reading this, I'd like to hear from you and hope that you could take some time to post a review on Amazon. Your feedback and support will help me to greatly improve my writing for future projects and make this book even better.

Your review is very important to me as it helps me morally. Hope this book helped you in some way to crack the exam.

Warm Regards,
Prof. Rita Carolyn